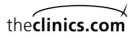
the**clinics.com**

VETERINARY CLINICS
OF NORTH AMERICA

Small Animal Practice

Respiratory Physiology, Diagnostics, and Disease

GUEST EDITOR
Lynelle R. Johnson, DVM, MS, PhD

September 2007 • Volume 37 • Number 5

SAUNDERS

An Imprint of Elsevier, Inc.
PHILADELPHIA   LONDON   TORONTO   MONTREAL   SYDNEY   TOKYO

W.B. SAUNDERS COMPANY
A Division of Elsevier Inc.

Elsevier, Inc., 1600 John F. Kennedy Blvd., Suite 1800, Philadelphia, PA 19103-2899

http://www.vetsmall.theclinics.com

VETERINARY CLINICS OF NORTH AMERICA:	Volume 37, Number 5
SMALL ANIMAL PRACTICE	ISSN 0195-5616
September 2007	ISBN-13: 978-1-4160-5139-8
Editor: John Vassallo; j.vassallo@elsevier.com	ISBN-10: 1-4160-5139-2

The ideas and opinions expressed in *Veterinary Clinics of North America: Small Animal Practice* do not necessarily reflect those of the Publisher. The Publisher does not assume any responsibility for any injury and/or damage to persons or property arising out of or related to any use of the material contained in this periodical. The reader is advised to check the appropriate medical literature and the product information currently provided by the manufacturer of each drug to be administered to verify the dosage, the method and duration of administration, or contraindications. It is the responsibility of the treating physician or other health care professional, relying on independent experience and knowledge of the patient, to determine drug dosages and the best treatment for the patient. Mention of any product in this issue should not be construed as endorsement by the contributors, editors, or the Publisher of the product or manufacturers' claims.

Veterinary Clinics of North America: Small Animal Practice (ISSN 0195-5616) is published bimonthly (For Post Office use only: volume 37 issue 5 of 6) by Elsevier Inc., 360 Park Avenue South, New York, NY 10010-1710. Months of issue are January, March, May, July, September, and November. Business and Editorial offices: 1600 John F. Kennedy Blvd., Suite 1800, Philadelphia, PA 19103-2899. Customer Service Office: 6277 Sea Harbor Drive, Orlando, FL 32887-4800. Periodicals postage paid at New York, NY and additional mailing offices. Subscription prices are $187.00 per year for US individuals, $297.00 per year for US institutions, $94.00 per year for US students and residents, $248.00 per year for Canadian individuals, $373.00 per year for Canadian institutions, $259.00 per year for international individuals, $373.00 per year for international institutions and $127.00 per year for Canadian and foreign students/residents. To receive student/resident rate, orders must be accompanied by name of affiliated institution, date of term, and the *signature* of program/residency coordinator on institution letterhead. Orders will be billed at individual rate until proof of status is received. Foreign air speed delivery is included in all *Clinics* subscription prices. All prices are subject to change without notice. **POSTMASTER**: Send address changes to *Veterinary Clinics of North America: Small Animal Practice*, Elsevier Periodicals Customer Service, 6277 Sea Harbor Drive, Orlando, FL 32887-4800, USA; phone: 1-800-654-2452 [toll free number for US customers], or (+1)(407) 345-4000 [customers outside US]; fax: (+1)(407) 363-1354; email: usjcs@elsevier.com.

Veterinary Clinics of North America: Small Animal Practice is also published in Japanese by Inter Zoo Publishing Co., Ltd., Aoyama Crystal-Bldg 5F, 3-5-12 Kitaaoyama, Minato-ku, Tokyo 107-0061, Japan.

Reprints: For copies of 100 or more, of articles in this publication, please contact the Commercial Reprints Department, Elsevier Inc., 360 Park Avenue South, New York, New York 10010-1710. Tel. (212) 633-3813 Fax: (212) 462-1935, email: reprints@elsevier.com.

Veterinary Clinics of North America: Small Animal Practice is covered in *Current Contents/Agriculture, Biology and Environmental Sciences, Science Citation Index, ASCA, Index Medicus, Excerpta Medica*, and *BIOSIS*.

Printed in the United States of America.

Respiratory Physiology, Diagnostics, and Disease

GUEST EDITOR

LYNELLE R. JOHNSON, DVM, MS, PhD, Diplomate, American College of Veterinary Internal Medicine; Associate Professor, Department of Medicine and Epidemiology, University of California at Davis, Davis, California

CONTRIBUTORS

JONATHAN F. BACH, DVM, Diplomate, American College of Veterinary Internal Medicine (Small Animal Medicine); Diplomate, American College of Veterinary Emergency and Critical Care; Assistant Professor, Department of Medical Sciences, University of Wisconsin School of Veterinary Medicine, Madison, Wisconsin

FIONA E. CAMPBELL, BVSc (Hons), MACVSc, PhD, Diplomate, American College of Veterinary Internal Medicine (Cardiology); Veterinary Medical Teaching Hospital, School of Veterinary Medicine, University of California at Davis, Davis, California; Veterinary Registrar (Cardiology), Veterinary Teaching Hospital, School of Veterinary Science, University of Queensland, St. Lucia, Queensland, Australia

SCOTT J. CAMPBELL, BVSc (Hons), MACVSc, Diplomate, American College of Veterinary Nutrition; WALTHAM Specialist in Clinical Nutrition, WALTHAM UCVMC-SD Clinical Nutrition Program, University of California Veterinary Medical Center–San Diego, San Diego, California

CÉCILE CLERCX, DVM, PhD, Diplomate, European College of Veterinary Internal Medicine-Companion Animals; Professor, Faculty of Veterinary Medicine, Department of Veterinary Clinical Sciences, Small Animal Internal Medicine, University of Liége, Liége, Belgium

LEAH A. COHN, DVM, PhD, Diplomate, American College of Veterinary Internal Medicine; Associate Professor, Department of Veterinary Medicine and Surgery, University of Missouri-Columbia College of Veterinary Medicine, Columbia, Missouri

ANDREW M. HOFFMAN, DVM, DVSc, Diplomate, American College of Veterinary Internal Medicine (Large Animal Internal Medicine); Associate Professor; and Director, Lung Foundation Testing Laboratory, Department of Clinical Sciences, Cummings School of Veterinary Medicine, Tufts University, North Grafton, Massachusetts

ERIC G. JOHNSON, DVM, Diplomate, American College of Veterinary Radiology; Assistant Professor, Department of Surgical and Radiological Sciences, School of Veterinary Medicine, Veterinary Medical Teaching Hospital Small Animal Clinic, University of California at Davis, Davis, California

CATRIONA M. MACPHAIL, DVM, PhD, Diplomate, American College of Veterinary Surgeons; Assistant Professor, Small Animal Soft Tissue Surgery, Department of Clinical Sciences, College of Veterinary Medicine and Biomedical Sciences, Colorado State University, Fort Collins, Colorado

CARRIE J. MILLER, DVM, Diplomate, American College of Veterinary Internal Medicine (Small Animal Internal Medicine); Staff Internist, Wheat Ridge Veterinary Specialists, Wheat Ridge, Colorado

DOMINIQUE PEETERS, DVM, PhD, Diplomate, European College of Veterinary Internal Medicine-Companion Animals; Senior Lecturer, Faculty of Veterinary Medicine, Department of Veterinary Clinical Sciences, Small Animal Internal Medicine, University of Liège, Liège, Belgium

CAROL R. REINERO, DVM, PhD, Diplomate, American College of Veterinary Internal Medicine; Assistant Professor, Department of Veterinary Medicine and Surgery, University of Missouri-Columbia College of Veterinary Medicine, Columbia, Missouri

ELIZABETH A. ROZANSKI, DVM, Diplomate, American College of Veterinary Internal Medicine (Small Animal Medicine); Diplomate, American College of Veterinary Emergency and Critical Care; Assistant Professor, Section of Critical Care, Department of Clinical Sciences, Cummings School of Veterinary Medicine, Tufts University, North Grafton, Massachusetts

SCOTT P. SHAW, DVM, Diplomate, American College of Veterinary Emergency and Critical Care; Section of Critical Care, Department of Clinical Sciences, Cummings School of Veterinary Medicine, Tufts University, North Grafton, Massachusetts

ERIK R. WISNER, DVM, Diplomate, American College of Veterinary Radiology; Professor; and Vice-Chair, Department of Surgical and Radiological Sciences; and Service Chief, Diagnostic Imaging, School of Veterinary Medicine, Veterinary Medical Teaching Hospital Small Animal Clinic, University of California at Davis, Davis, California

Respiratory Physiology, Diagnostics, and Disease

Advances in Respiratory Imaging 879

Eric G. Johnson and Erik R. Wisner

Although conventional radiography is still the first diagnostic imaging approach to respiratory disease, CT is proving to be invaluable as an adjunctive procedure in characterizing nasal and thoracic pathologic findings. CT eliminates superimposition of overlying structures and offers superior contrast resolution as compared with conventional radiography. These advantages allow for more precise characterization and localization of lesions and are invaluable for guiding rhinoscopic, bronchoscopic, and surgical procedures.

Update on Canine Sinonasal Aspergillosis 901

Dominique Peeters and Cécile Clercx

Sinonasal aspergillosis is a frequent cause of nasal discharge that occurs in otherwise healthy, young to middle-aged dogs. A local immune dysfunction is suspected in affected animals, and the role of increased interleukin-10 mRNA expression in the nasal mucosa of affected dogs is currently under investigation. Despite recent advances in imaging techniques, the "gold standard" for diagnosing the disease is direct visualization of fungal plaques during endoscopy or observation of fungal elements on cytology or histopathologic examination. Treatment can be challenging; however, the use of topical enilconazole or clotrimazole through noninvasive techniques has increased the success of treatment and decreased the morbidity and duration of hospitalization.

Canine Eosinophilic Bronchopneumopathy 917

Cécile Clercx and Dominique Peeters

Eosinophilic bronchopneumopathy (EBP) is a disease characterized by eosinophilic infiltration of the lung and bronchial mucosa, as demonstrated by examination of bronchoalveolar lavage fluid cytologic preparations or histologic examination of the bronchial mucosa. Although the precise cause of EBP is unknown, a hypersensitivity to aeroallergens is suspected. The diagnosis relies on typical history and clinical signs, demonstration of bronchopulmonary eosinophilia by cytology or histopathologic examination, and exclusion of known causes of lower airway eosinophilia. Most dogs display an excellent response to oral corticosteroid therapy; however, side effects of this treatment can be limiting. New therapeutic approaches are being studied, including the use of aerosol therapy, cyclosporine, or drugs interfering with T helper 2 immune response.

Interstitial Lung Diseases 937

Carol R. Reinero and Leah A. Cohn

Several noninfectious nonneoplastic interstitial lung diseases (ILDs) have been recognized in dogs and cats. Overall, these ILDs are poorly characterized in dogs and cats, although awareness of the conditions based on descriptions of clinical case series may be increasing. Lung biopsy remains crucial to the diagnosis, characterization, and classification of ILDs. Histopathologic findings can help to guide clinicians in selecting appropriate therapy and providing an accurate prognosis to pet owners. Only with definitive recognition of these pulmonary conditions can our knowledge of the clinical course and response to therapy be improved.

Pulmonary hypertension (PHT) is the primary cardiac consequence of pulmonary disease. It develops as alveolar hypoxia of pulmonary disease, coupled with vasoactive and mitogenic substances released from pulmonary endothelial and vascular smooth muscle cells damaged by the primary disease process, mediates arterial vasoconstriction and vascular remodeling to raise pulmonary vascular resistance. Independent of the underlying pulmonary disease, PHT produces clinical signs of respiratory distress, exercise intolerance, syncope, and right heart failure. Diagnosis of PHT is made by estimation of pulmonary artery pressures by means of continuous-wave Doppler echocardiographic assessment of tricuspid or pulmonic regurgitant flow velocity. Treatment of PHT is directed at the underlying pulmonary disease but may also aim to attenuate pulmonary artery pressure and limit the clinical sequelae of PHT. No treatments are of proven benefit in veterinary patients; irrespective of the nature of the inciting pulmonary disease, the prognosis is often grave.

Effective respiratory therapy depends on obtaining a definitive diagnosis and following established recommendations for treatment. Unfortunately, many respiratory conditions are idiopathic in origin or are attributable to nonspecific inflammation. In some situations, disorders are controlled rather than cured. Recent advances in pulmonary therapeutics include the use of new agents to treat common diseases and application of local delivery of drugs to enhance drug effect and minimize side effects.

Pyothorax is the accumulation of septic suppurative inflammation within the pleural cavity. The cause and source of infection in dogs and cats often are unknown. Management of these cases can be challenging, because controversy exists over the best method for treatment. Reported outcomes and recurrence rates vary widely.

Nutritional Considerations for Animals with Pulmonary Disease

Scott J. Campbell

Recent publications in the human and veterinary literature have indicated that patients with pulmonary disease require specific nutritional consideration to ensure that optimal benefit is derived with nutrition support. Although additional research is needed in this area, preliminary recommendations can be made using information from the scant studies performed thus far in veterinary medicine and from information extrapolated from the human literature. These recommendations are likely to provide significant clinical benefit to patients with pulmonary disease. This article aims to provide the reader with a summary of the available information and links to other relevant sources.

FORTHCOMING ISSUES

RECENT ISSUES

Preface

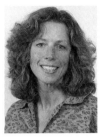

Lynelle R. Johnson, DVM, MS, PhD

Guest Editor

Upper and lower respiratory tract diseases are encountered commonly in small animal practice and often represent both a diagnostic and therapeutic challenge. A thorough physical examination is helpful in localizing disease to a particular region within the respiratory tract. Knowledge of the etiology and pathophysiology of disease assists the clinician in formulating an accurate diagnostic plan. Ultimately, effective treatment depends on determining the cause and severity of respiratory dysfunction.

This issue brings together a number of talented individuals in the disciplines of medicine, radiology, and surgery to provide a comprehensive update on important issues in respiratory medicine. The first articles in this issue reinforce the relevant physiology and immunology of the respiratory tract that are needed to understand clinical manifestations of disease and to recognize infectious, inflammatory, and structural diseases in respiratory patients. Articles on physical examination, cardiopulmonary interactions, respiratory therapy, and nutrition for the respiratory patient provide pearls of wisdom for both diagnostic testing and clinical management. A comprehensive article on diagnostic imaging nicely demonstrates the complementary roles of radiology and computed tomography in the diagnosis of respiratory disease. Finally, specific articles on challenging infectious and inflammatory diseases of the upper and lower respiratory tract illustrate the value of combining scientific research and clinical medicine to improve animal health.

This issue of *Veterinary Clinics of North America: Small Animal Practice* will serve as a valuable source of information in the years to come. Many thanks to the contributing authors, many of whom have expanded our knowledge of respiratory tract diseases with their efforts in research and through participation in the Veterinary Comparative Respiratory Society. Special thanks to my

0195-5616/07/$ – see front matter
doi:10.1016/j.cvsm.2007.06.002
vetsmall.theclinics.com

mentor and friend, Dr. Brendan McKiernan, who continues to teach me everything I know.

Lynelle R. Johnson, DVM, MS, PhD
Department of Medicine and Epidemiology
2108 Tupper Hall
University of California at Davis
One Shields Avenue
Davis, CA 95616, USA

E-mail address: lrjohnson@ucdavis.edu

Airway Physiology and Clinical Function Testing

Andrew M. Hoffman, DVM, DVSc

Lung Foundation Testing Laboratory, Department of Clinical Sciences,
Cummings School of Veterinary Medicine, Tufts University, Room 110, Building 21,
200 Westboro Road, North Grafton, MA 01536, USA

UPPER AIRWAY PHYSIOLOGY RELATED TO AIRWAY DISORDERS

The upper airways are composed of the nasal cavities, nasopharynx, and glottis. These structures play a crucial role in the defense of the distal airways from cooling, desiccation, and bombardment with particles. Underscoring their significant contribution, bypass of the upper airways by endotracheal intubation and insufflation of dry air evoke epithelial injury, airway remodeling, inflammation, and hyperreactivity in canine subjects [1–3]. Large cavernous venous plexuses in the turbinates, sinuses, and septum serve the purpose of counteracting these potentially harmful effects of the environment by heating inspired gas, which is further humidified in the lung. The venous plexuses are divided functionally and anatomically into anterior and posterior collection systems [4,5]. Vascular filling is largely determined by venous capacitance (storage capacity) and tone (constriction) in the outflow vasculature. The anterior plexuses drain through the dorsal nasal and anterior collecting veins, and the posterior plexuses empty by way of the lateral and septal collecting veins and the sphenopalatine vein (caudally), with final drainage into the external jugular vein. The anterior plexuses (right and left) communicate through the dorsal nasal veins across the bridge of the anterior nose. The balance between the effects of parasympathetic and sympathetic agonists on inflow or outflow of the nasal veins dictates whether decongestion or congestion predominates. Simultaneous stimulation of the parasympathetic and sympathetic nervous supply results in sympathetic dominance [6]. The α_1 and α_2 adrenoceptors mediate decreased venous capacitance, with dominance by α_2 receptors, whereas venous dilation is mediated equally by β_1 and β_2 adrenoceptors, with the combined effect of reducing nasal resistance (ie, decongestion) [7]. Interestingly, acetylcholine (Ach) causes decongestion at high concentrations and congestion at low doses. In the dog, this is

E-mail address: andrew.hoffman@tufts.edu

0195-5616/07/$ – see front matter
doi:10.1016/j.cvsm.2007.05.013

apparently attributable to specific constriction of the posterior outflow veins (lateral and septal collecting veins) only at higher concentrations; lower concentrations cause nitric-oxide–dependent relaxation [8].

The upper airways contribute to most air flow resistance of the respiratory tract. Deformities of the upper airways therefore have substantial consequences to air flow. In brachycephalic syndrome (BCS), soft palate elongation and thickening contribute to air flow limitation [9]. In approximately half of affected dogs, there is restriction in the cross-sectional area of the nares and nasal turbinates, furthering the need to generate negative pressure to overcome the inspiratory flow limitation. The breathing pattern in BCS exemplifies the effects of airway resistance (R_{aw}): paradoxic movement of the abdominal and rib cage components. The heightened negative pressure required to overcome stenotic nasal passages and soft palate disorders may secondarily promote eversion of laryngeal saccules, worsening airway obstruction. English Bulldogs with BCS show marked sleepiness in comparison to normal dogs [10]. Obesity, as in human beings, may worsen upper airway obstruction, although the exact link is unclear. As is also the case in people, airway obstruction is much more apparent during sleep. Airway obstruction during sleep in the Bulldog coincides with periods of rapid eye movement (REM) that normally suppress muscle activity. In the normal dog, no muscle activity is required to maintain pharyngeal patency; however, in the Bulldog, the loss of pharyngeal dilator activity allows the pharynx to collapse [11]. Collapse of the pharynx tends to occur at end-expiration in the Bulldog [12], in contrast to normal dogs, in which fluctuations in patency favor opening during expiration. As time goes on, airway obstruction with BCS worsens because of repeated injury to the pharyngeal muscles and consequent edema and fibrosis of these muscle groups [13,14]. The significance of nasal and soft palate abnormalities air flow to airway obstruction and hypersomnolence is exemplified by the improvement seen in many dogs with BCS that undergo nares or palatal resection or sacculectomy, however.

Laryngeal paralysis is a common cause for mild, moderate, or severe respiratory distress in older large-breed dogs that causes distinct inspiratory flow limitation [15]. The glottis is innervated by branches of cranial nerve X. Patency of the glottic opening is largely a function of positioning of the arytenoid cartilages, which are abducted by the cricoarytenoideus dorsalis (CAD) muscles. These are ipsilaterally innervated by the caudal laryngeal nerves (distal branches of recurrent laryngeal nerve). Damage or degeneration of the recurrent laryngeal nerve or CAD muscle results in ipsilateral laryngeal paresis or paralysis. In contrast to horses, clinical signs of laryngeal disease in dogs are typically only observed with bilateral paralysis. Although classic laryngeal paralysis causes an increase in airway resistance (R_{aw}) during inspiration, the addition of arytenoid edema, inflammation, or fibrosis can promote a "fixed" airway obstruction. Flow limitation may also reduce the efficiency of body cooling because of decreased air flow across the tongue, causing a vicious cycle of increased demand for ventilation and airway obstruction.

LOWER AIRWAY PHYSIOLOGY RELATED TO AIRWAY NARROWING (BRONCHOCONSTRICTION)

The lower airways consist of the trachea, bronchi, and bronchioles. Airway narrowing is the event that attracts the most attention of veterinarians. To understand the pathophysiology of airway narrowing better, it is worth considering the autonomic innervation and reflexes that control bronchoconstriction and bronchodilation. The distal airways (bronchi and bronchioles) are innervated by parasympathetic postganglionic nerves that use Ach for bronchoconstriction and by additional noncholinergic nonadrenergic (NANC) parasympathetic nerves that use vasoactive intestinal peptide (VIP) and nitric oxide for smooth muscle relaxation and bronchodilation [16]. In cats, the intrapulmonary airways (apart from the trachea) are richly innervated by noradrenergic (sympathetic) nerves causing smooth muscle relaxation, which are less prominent in the dog, although sympathetic stimulation causes bronchodilation in both species by means of β-adrenergic receptors on bronchial smooth muscle.

There is a certain amount of basal parasympathetic tone in bronchial smooth muscle that is abolished when the afferent vagal nerve endings (embedded in bronchial smooth muscle) are inhibited, for example, by topical application of lidocaine. These afferents are the sensory end of an important reflex arc (afferent, brain, and efferent pre- and postganglionic cholinergic) that leads to bronchoconstriction. This reflex arc can be blocked at the sensory end (using lidocaine) or efferent end (using atropine or topical anticholinergics) [17], as is customary before bronchoscopy in some cases. The efferent receptor with greatest relevance to airway function is the M_3 (muscarinic) receptor on bronchial or bronchiolar smooth muscle, where stimulation causes bronchoconstriction, mucus secretion, and bronchial arterial vasodilation. The M_1 receptor may facilitate this transmission; therefore, newer bronchodilators (eg, tiotropium bromide) are M_3/M_1 selective. For the clinician, it is important to recognize that a variety of stimuli to the airway surface initiate the bronchoconstrictive reflex arc, including mechanical (eg, bronchoscopy, particulates) and chemical-paracrine (eg, acid, histamine, secretions) factors, dynamic lung inflation, pulmonary edema, pulmonary embolism, and pneumothorax [17].

Due to the overwhelming influence of parasympathetic reflexes, the role of adrenergic nerves in the lower airways is minimal. Adrenoreceptors on airway smooth muscle are prevalent, however, and respond readily to circulating adrenaline or topical application of sympathomimetics. Stimulation of adrenoreceptors causes smooth muscle relaxation and bronchodilation (β_2) or bronchoconstriction (β_1). Bronchodilators (eg, albuterol, salmeterol) are strongly selective for β_2 receptors but possess some β_1 properties that can evoke undesirable side effects when overdosed (tachycardia).

AIRWAY FUNCTION TESTING

Traditional methods for diagnosing respiratory disease include physical examination, radiography, CT, arterial blood gases, bronchoscopy, and sampling of respiratory secretions, but these tests may still leave the clinician perplexed as to the origin of disease and the degree of respiratory embarrassment associated with the abnormal breathing pattern, recurrent cough, or exercise intolerance. Assessment of respiratory function is sometimes a more direct route to solving these questions. The value of pulmonary function testing (PFT) is (1) to confirm the suspicion regarding the pathophysiology of disease and (2) to uncover complex (multifactorial) factors that contribute to apparent signs. Indeed, what one learns from PFT is that the traditional "dichotomous" categorizations of obstructive versus restrictive, upper airway versus lower airway, or mechanical versus gas exchange problem are oversimplified. Veterinary patients exhibit dysfunction in multiple segments of the respiratory system, which interact or sum to produce clinical signs.

Generation of Air Flow

Air flow arises from voluntary and involuntary signals that drive muscular effort to expand the chest by (1) rib cage expansion and (2) caudal displacement of the diaphragm (Fig. 1). During inspiration, expansion of the chest shifts pleural pressure to a more negative value. Pleural pressure is often cited as the driving force to overcome elastic recoil and resistance (ie, respiratory system impedance). When pleural pressure descends to a more negative value (eg, from -2 to -7 cm H_2O), alveolar gas within the lung expands. Air flows into the lung down its pressure gradient but ceases to flow once alveolar pressure returns to zero (atmospheric pressure) at peak inspiration. Flow

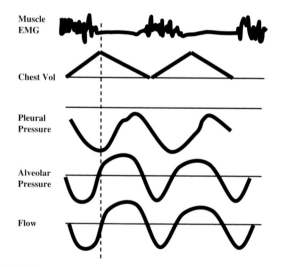

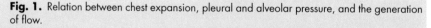

Fig. 1. Relation between chest expansion, pleural and alveolar pressure, and the generation of flow.

then reverses during expiration because of transient positive alveolar pressure created by elastic recoil, a process that does not require muscular effort at rest. At end-expiration, alveolar pressure returns to baseline and flow comes to a halt again. In sum, flow is directly attributable to fluctuations in alveolar pressure relative to atmospheric pressure that cycle from negative to positive during each breath. Hence, the appearance of alveolar pressure and flow waveforms (on a strip-chart) are superimposable, and inspiratory flow is often depicted in the negative direction to correspond with negative alveolar pressure. The relevance of alveolar pressure to flow is most important in discussion of the measurement of R_{aw}.

Flow Limitation

Causes of air flow limitation other than from reduced effort include loss of elastic recoil, airway narrowing, or nonlaminar flow (turbulence). The expected consequences of flow limitation (versus restriction of lung) are summarized in Table 1. Flow limitation may occur during inspiration or expiration or transiently during subsegments of inspiration (eg, laryngeal paralysis, tracheal collapse) or expiration (bronchial collapse). Flow restriction is created by the presence of a transmural pressure gradient that results in generation of a more negative pressure within the collapsing airway lumen relative to the surrounding alveoli. The choke point (point of narrowing) is determined by the temporal and spatial positioning of the maximum transmural pressure. Because the small airways (bronchioles) are unsupported by cartilage, and therefore rely on the surrounding alveolar parenchyma for tethering, they are a common site of dynamic airway narrowing, resulting in flow limitation. Certain activities, such as coughing, exercise, vomiting, abdominal pressure, and gastroesophageal reflux, have the potential to increase the transmural pressure gradient, promoting collapse of a segment of airway. Protective measures that counterbalance airway narrowing include parenchymal tethering of the bronchioles and cartilage that surround bronchi. These protective mechanisms fail in diseases such as bronchiectasis, tracheal injury or malformation, or emphysema, and the "wave" of transmural pressure favors narrowing of airways.

Measurement of Flow Limitation

Irrespective of the cause of dynamic airway narrowing, the net result is a demonstrable drop in flow during a particular segment of the breath, which is quantifiable at the airway opening using "spirometry" (the measurement of flow in and out of the respiratory system). Also accompanying flow limitation is a sharp increase in R_{aw}. Spirometry can be performed using a calibrated pneumotachograph or handheld spirometer. Although the handheld spirometer can provide expired or minute volumes, a pneumotachograph permits the measurement of flow rates and duration of breath segments (inspiratory and expiratory times). Most pneumotachographs are flow resistors that create a measurable pressure drop across their elements, which is linearly proportional to flow over

Table 1
Spirometry in small companion animals (dogs and cats) and typical effects of airway obstruction or restrictive disorders

Parameter	Abbreviation	Units	Instrument	Awake[a]	Effect of airway obstruction[b]	Effect of restriction[b]
Tidal volume	V_T	mL	Pneumotachograph	Yes	None or decrease	Decrease
Frequency	F	Breaths per minute	Pneumotachograph	Yes	None or decrease	Increase
Minute volume (expired)	V_E	mL	Pneumotachograph	Yes	None or decrease	None or decrease
Peak inspiratory flow	PIF	mL/s	Pneumotachograph	Yes	Decrease	Increase
Peak expiratory flow	PEF	mL/s	Pneumotachograph	Yes	Decrease	Increase
Inspiratory time	Ti	Second	Pneumotachograph	Yes	Increase with inspiratory obstruction	Decrease
Expiratory time	Te	Second	Pneumotachograph	Yes	Increase with expiratory obstruction	Decrease
Inspiratory capacity	IC	mL	Pneumotachograph, WBP	No	None	Decrease
Vital capacity	VC	mL	Pneumotachograph, WBP	No	None or decrease	Decrease
Total lung capacity	TLC	mL	Pneumotachograph, WBP	No	None or decrease	Decrease
Functional residual capacity	FRC_{He}	mL	Helium dilution	Yes	Decrease (artifact)[c]	Decrease
	FRC_{pleth}		WBP	No	None or increase	Decrease
Residual volume	RV	mL	WBP	No	None or increase	Decrease

Abbreviations: pleth, plethysmography; WBP, whole-body plethysmography.
[a] Measurements that can be made without anesthesia.
[b] Typical findings.
[c] Helium does not communicate with trapped gas; thus, FRC_{He} underestimates actual FRC.

a prescribed range. Pneumotachographs are coupled with a face mask for collection of flow. Technically speaking, one needs pressure tubing, a low-flow differential pressure transducer, an amplifier, a digitizer (A-to-D card), and data acquisition software to make these measurements. Because of the expense of these systems, they are largely found in research laboratories. In accordance with the trend in human medicine, however, increased availability and decreased cost are expected in the near future.

In human medicine, the detection of expiratory flow limitation is enhanced by asking the patient to exhale forcefully to increase transmural pressure and promote airway closure. This technique can be used in intubated animals, and measurements during natural breathing but not forced breathing are feasible in the unanesthetized small animal patient. There are advantages to addressing air flow during tidal breathing, because signs of flow limitation are more likely to be clinically relevant (more specific). Tidal breathing can be enhanced by temporary exposure of the patient to carbon dioxide (CO_2) [18] or more simply, by inducing respirations within a dead space [19], resulting in doubling or tripling of peak flows. The induced hyperpnea amplifies transmural pressure, and therefore exacerbates flow limitation whether it is intrathoracic or extrathoracic. The effectiveness of hyperpnea in unmasking pathologic conditions is evidenced by the utility of doxapram (2.2 mg/kg administered intravenously) to facilitate laryngoscopic examination of canine subjects [20].

CLINICAL AIRWAY FUNCTION TESTING

Air flow limitation is a highly prevalent problem in small animals; examples include canine laryngeal paralysis, tracheal stenosis (collapse?), bronchial collapse, and feline bronchopulmonary disease ("asthma"). Loss of elastic recoil (eg, emphysema) also imparts airway obstruction as a result of failure to tether open the bronchioles, but emphysema is rare in domestic animals [21]. Airway obstruction is associated with increased work of breathing, hypoxemia, and hypercapnia if ventilation is compromised. The breathing pattern may show prolongation of inspiratory or expiratory time and asynchrony between the rib cage and diaphragm (ie, abdomen). Airway obstruction is best quantified by the measurement of resistance. The physical basis for resistance is the loss of kinetic energy attributable to friction of air traveling through narrowed airways. Turbulence, or nonlaminar flow, compounds this frictional (viscous) loss of pressure. The greater the resistance, the greater is the pressure drop between segments of the airway. Nonuniformity of bronchoconstriction also contributes to resistance [22]. Determinants of resistance within a defined segment of the respiratory tract are (1) driving pressure and (2) flow. Indeed, the relation between driving pressure and flow can be expressed as follows:

$$\text{Resistance} = \delta\,\text{Pressure}/\delta\,\text{Flow} = \delta P/\delta V'$$

Table 2
Measurement of resistance (cm H_2O/L/s) in conscious animals requires continuous measurement across the segment of interest while measuring flow

Resistance	Abbreviation	Flow	P_1	P_2	Possible site(s) of obstruction
Airway resistance	R_{aw}	Mask	Mask	Alveolus	Upper or lower airways
Upper airway resistance	R_{Uaw}	Mask	Mask	Trachea	Nasal, pharyngeal, laryngeal
Pulmonary resistance	R_L	Mask	Mask/ET	Pleural esophageal	Upper airways, lower airways, lung parenchyma
Respiratory system	R_{RS}	ET	ET	Atmosphere	Airways, lung, or chest wall

Abbreviations: ET, endotracheal tube; mask, face mask; P_1, proximal pressure sensor; P_2, distal pressure sensor.

Resistance in this formula is expressed generically (ie, without specification of the anatomic segment of interest). To localize resistance, a more specific "address" is needed, for example:

Airway Resistance = δ Alveolar Pressure/δ Flow

or

$$R_{aw} = \delta P_{alv}/\delta V'$$

This additional level of complexity is valuable because it specifies the site of airway narrowing that is being investigated. For example, if one can isolate resistance to the airways, the contribution of the parenchyma (tissue resistance) can be eliminated. An alternative approach is to lump together airway and parenchymal contributions to resistance (Airways + Tissue Resistance = Pulmonary Resistance [R_L]):

Pulmonary Resistance = δ Transpulmonary Pressure/δ Flow

or

$$R_L = \delta P_{pl}/\delta V'$$

Hence, the sites of pressure measurement are proximal and distal to the segment where resistance is measured. The terminologies used to describe different types of resistance and sites where pressure probes are used to generate these variables are shown in Table 2. In most cases, the reference probe (pressure 1 [P_1]) is open to the atmosphere, the face mask, or distally beyond the end of an endotracheal tube (to bypass tube resistance). The distal site of pressure measurement (P_2) largely determines the segment over which resistance is to be measured.

Tidal Breathing Flow-Volume Loops

Perhaps the simplest technique to discern flow limitation is by means of use of a pneumotachograph to record flow versus time to construct a flow-volume loop using a data acquisition system. The pneumotachograph is calibrated using known flows or volumes drawn through the device and then applied by means of a face mask to the patient. Several variables can be obtained (Table 3) that can be used to characterize flow limitation, such as peak flows (peak expiratory flow [PEF] and peak inspiratory flow [PIF]), flow at 25% or 75% of exhaled volume, or simply midtidal expiratory flow (EF_{50}) [23], with the latter widely used in rodent species during bronchial challenges [24]. McKiernan and Johnson [18] reviewed the utility of tidal breathing flow-volume loops in dogs, and McKiernan and colleagues reviewed that in cats [25].

In more severe airway obstruction, such as laryngeal paralysis, chronic bronchitis with tracheal collapse, or pharyngeal masses, flow limitation is easily detectable using tidal breathing flow-volume loops [23,25]. One of the drawbacks of using flow or flow-volume loops for analysis of airway obstruction is a lack of sensitivity. In one study, Bedenice and colleagues [19] found that flow-derived variables lacked sensitivity for mild to moderate fixed or dynamic upper airway obstruction (simulated experimentally using external resistive loads) in comparison to specific airway resistance (sR_{aw}) in dogs. The lower sensitivity of flow-volume loops compared with body plethysmography is also evident in human beings [26]. As a result, airway obstruction with clinical relevance (eg, bronchial narrowing) may be missed using flow-derived measurements alone. Sensitivity of flow-derived measurements during tidal breathing has been augmented in people using the negative expiratory pressure (NEP) method, whereby a negative pressure is imposed on the patient's airway to promote airway closure in affected (but not in normal) patients. The NEP method has not been fully explored in small animals, however.

Measurement of Specific Airway Resistance Using Head-Out Plethysmography in Dogs and Cats

In human patients, R_{aw} is traditionally measured using whole-body plethysmography. Determination of R_{aw} entails separate measurements of sR_{aw} and functional residual capacity (FRC). sR_{aw} is the product of R_{aw} and FRC (R_{aw} [cm $H_2O/L/s$] · FRC in L = sR_{aw} [cm/s]); therefore, R_{aw} is computed as sR_{aw}/FRC. The plethysmographic measurement of FRC in conscious animals is problematic because of the requirement of airway occlusion (met with displeasure by dogs and cats), but it is feasible to measure sR_{aw}. An increase in R_{aw} (airway narrowing) or an increase in FRC (air trapping or hyperinflation) can contribute to an increase in sR_{aw}. Asthma is an example of a condition that causes R_{aw} and FRC to increase (with air trapping), causing sR_{aw} to increase to a greater extent than R_{aw} or FRC. Alternately, fixed

Table 3
Methods to quantify airway obstruction in small animal patients

Method	Variable	Symbol	Units	Awake	Airway obstruction
Pneumotachography	Peak flow	PEF, PIF	mL/s	Yes	Decrease
Pneumotachography	Flow at, for example, 50% tidal volume	EF_{50}	mL/s	Yes	Decrease
Forced expiratory maneuver	Forced expiratory flow	$FEF_x{}^a$	mL/s	No	Decrease
	Forced expiratory volume	$FEV_x{}^a$	mL	No	Decrease
Classic mechanics (esophageal balloon method)	Pulmonary resistance	R_L	cm H_2O/mL/s	No	Increase
Interrupter method	Dynamic compliance	C_{dyn}	mL/cm H_2O	No	Decrease
	Respiratory system resistance	R_{RS}	cm H_2O/mL/s	No	Increase
Impulse oscillometry	Respiratory system resistance	R_{RS}	cm H_2O/mL/s	Yes	Increase
	Respiratory system resistance	R_{RS}	cm H_2O/mL/s	No	Increase
Forced oscillatory mechanics	Airway resistance	R_{aw}	cm H_2O/mL/s	No	Increase
	Tissue resistance	G_{ti}	cm H_2O/mL/s	No	Increase
Unrestrained whole-body plethysmography	Enhanced pause	Penh	Unitless	Yes	Increase
Head-out plethysmography	Specific airway resistance	sR_{aw}	cm $H_2O \times s$	Yes	Increase

^{a}x, percentage of exhaled volume specified by investigator for end point of measurement (eg, 25%, 50%, or 75%).

obstructions of the large airways increase R_{aw} but may have no effect on FRC. Another useful feature of sR_{aw} is that it is largely independent of body size, because FRC is scaled somewhat to body size. This assumption, may be challenged, however, as different breeds are shown to have different FRCs per body weight (eg, 44 mL/kg in awake Beagles [27] and 120 mL/kg in Greyhounds [28]).

One solution to measurement of sR_{aw} in conscious unsedated dogs was recently advanced by Bedenice and colleagues [19,29]. Head-out whole-body plethysmography (HOP) is a modification of whole-body plethysmography originally described for human beings by Dubois and colleagues [30].This technique permits measurement of sR_{aw} and spirometry simultaneously and is well tolerated with little or no prior experience by the patient in most (>90%) canine patients. The canine patient is led into a plexiglass box (300 L) through a rear door and is coaxed to sit toward the front of the box, where the head projects through a large opening (Fig. 2). A door for the head region is closed around the head by way of a rubber shroud, derived from the neck-head portion of a dry scuba suit. A face mask is applied to the muzzle and connected to a calibrated pneumotachograph. The pneumotachograph is connected by means of a short length of tube back to the box so that the dog is effectively breathing as if totally within the box. To measure sR_{aw}, volumetric changes derived by measuring box pressure and flow at the mask are recorded concurrently and plotted on X-Y coordinates (Fig. 3). The left side of the polygon represents the transition between expiration and inspiration, where gas is preconditioned to body temperature and pressure standard to avoid distortion of plethysmographic measurements of volume attributable to heating and

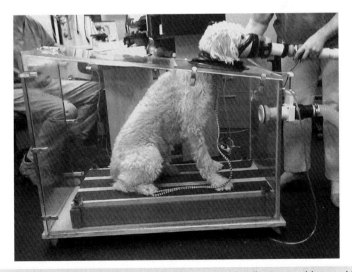

Fig. 2. Head-out whole-body plethysmography in a Labradoodle (1-year-old spayed female).

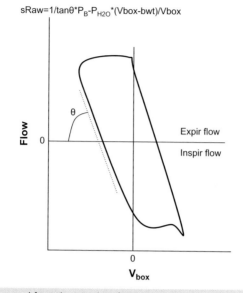

$$sRaw = 1/tan\theta * P_B - P_{H2O} * (Vbox-bwt)/Vbox$$

Fig. 3. sR_{aw} is computed from the X-Y plot of Vbox and Flow as follows: $sR_{aw} = (1/tan\theta) \times (P_B - P_{H2O}) \times (Vbox - bw/Vbox)$.

humidification of inspired air [31,32]. The angle (θ) measured from the left side of the X-Y polygon is used to compute sR_{aw}:

$$sR_{aw} = 1/tan\theta \times (P_B - P_{H2O}) \times Cf \times (Vbox - bwt)/Vbox$$

where θ is the angle converted to radians, $P_B - P_{H2O}$ is atmospheric minus water vapor pressures in cm H_2O, Cf relates the units on the X axis to the Y axis in terms of centimeters of paper size, Vbox is the internal volume of the plethysmograph, and bwt is the body weight of animal. Normal reference values were obtained for sR_{aw} (10.1 ± 2.8 cm $H_2O \times$s) and R_{aw} (4.6 ± 1.9 cm H_2O/L/s) [19]. Body condition score influences sR_{aw} and R_{aw} positively, such that moderate obesity (condition score 7–8) doubles sR_{aw} [33]. The change is observed most readily while the dog is hyperpneic. The mechanism is unknown but seems to be independent of body condition effects on FRC.

Clinical examples of loops derived from HOP in dogs are demonstrated in Fig. 4. Dogs are routinely tested during quiet breathing and hyperpnea, with the latter produced by breathing in the connector tube to cause rebreathing of CO_2 to some extent. There is no effect of hyperpnea or tachypnea (panting, case A) on sR_{aw} in normal dogs [19]; similarly, panting versus quiet tidal breathing showed no effect on sR_{aw} in human beings [31]. Smoking caused an increase in baseline sR_{aw} in some cases (eg, case B). The acute effects of cigarette smoke on dogs seem to be most profound in the peripheral (versus central) airway and seem to involve stimulation of nicotinic parasympathetic

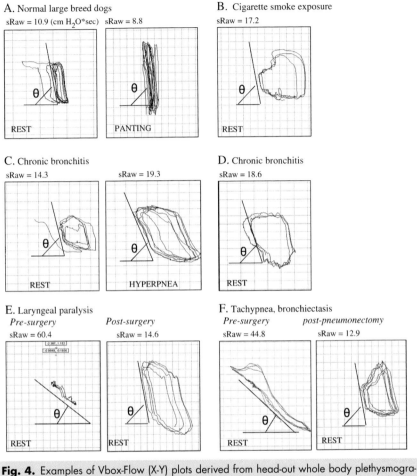

A. Normal large breed dogs
sRaw = 10.9 (cm H$_2$O*sec) sRaw = 8.8

REST   PANTING

B. Cigarette smoke exposure
sRaw = 17.2

REST

C. Chronic bronchitis
sRaw = 14.3   sRaw = 19.3

REST   HYPERPNEA

D. Chronic bronchitis
sRaw = 18.6

REST

E. Laryngeal paralysis
Pre-surgery   *Post-surgery*
sRaw = 60.4   sRaw = 14.6

REST   REST

F. Tachypnea, bronchiectasis
Pre-surgery   *post-pneumonectomy*
sRaw = 44.8   sRaw = 12.9

REST   REST

Fig. 4. Examples of Vbox-Flow (X-Y) plots derived from head-out whole body plethysmography. The X axis is Vbox (volumetric shift created by changes in alveolar pressure), and the Y axis is pneumotachographic flow (inspiration negative).

receptors in that species [34]. Chronic tobacco smoke exposure produced airway remodeling in Beagle dogs [35], but the effects of environmental (passive) tobacco smoke on airway function in dogs are unknown. Chronic bronchitis was evidenced by a mild to moderate increase in sR$_{aw}$ (cases C and D) that was worsened by hyperpnea (case C). Laryngeal paralysis caused a dramatic increase in sR$_{aw}$ that seemed to be alleviated by surgery (eg, arytenoid lateralization in case E) [19]. Focal bronchiectasis characterized by marked respiratory distress was associated with elevated sR$_{aw}$ in one case that was reduced by lung lobectomy (case F). In the future, measurement of sR$_{aw}$ may offer a sensitive noninvasive method to characterize subtle airway dysfunction in outpatients. The visual assessment of plethysmographic loops is extremely helpful to examine the fixed versus dynamic and inspiratory versus expiratory characteristics of airway obstruction. The value of this approach is exemplified by the more than 50 years of continuous application in PFT laboratories in human patients. The effects of surgery or medical interventions can be monitored over time, giving objective evidence that procedures are improving airway function at rest and during moderate hyperpnea.

SUMMARY

Although there are significant advances in PFT in small animals, the transition to clinical practice has been slow. The link to clinical practice is usually commercialization; thus, the field awaits the availability of inexpensive PFT systems for veterinary practice. Such systems are currently available for equine and laboratory animal testing, and canine-feline systems are expected to be developed in the near future. With the availability and use of PFT, the pathophysiology of airway dysfunction should be better understood by association of airway mechanics with functional (arterial blood gases), structural (imaging, histologic, and bronchoscopic), and cytologic outcomes. The addition of PFT should enhance our understanding of airway disorders in small animals and lead to more sophisticated subgrouping of conditions involving all levels of the airways.

References

[1] Davis MS, Freed AN. Repeated hyperventilation causes peripheral airways inflammation, hyperreactivity, and impaired bronchodilation in dogs. Am J Respir Crit Care Med 2001; 164:785–9.

[2] Davis MS, Freed AN. Repetitive hyperpnoea causes peripheral airway obstruction and eosinophilia. Eur Respir J 1999;14:57–62.

[3] Davis MS, Schofield B, Freed AN. Repeated peripheral airway hyperpnea causes inflammation and remodeling in dogs. Med Sci Sports Exerc 2003;35:608–16.

[4] Lung MA, Wang JC. Arterial supply, venous drainage and collateral circulation in the nose of the anaesthetized dog. J Phys 1987;391:57–70.

[5] Wang JC, Lung MA. Nasal venous drainage in the dog. Rhinology 1987;25:13–6.

[6] Lung MA, Wang JC. Autonomic nervous control of nasal vasculature and airflow resistance in the anaesthetized dog. J Phys 1989;419:121–39.

[7] Wang M, Lung MA. Adrenergic mechanisms in canine nasal venous systems. Br J Pharmacol 2003;138:145–55.

[8] Wang M, Lung MA. Acetylcholine induces contractile and relaxant effects in canine nasal venous systems. Eur Respir J 2006;28:839–46.

[9] Lorison DBR, White RAS. Brachycephalic airway obstructive syndrome: a review of 118 cases. Canine Pract 1997;22:18–21.

[10] Hendricks JC, Kline LR, Kovalski RJ, et al. The English bulldog: a natural model of sleep-disordered breathing. J Appl Physiol 1987;63:1344–50.

[11] Hendricks JC, Petrof BJ, Panckeri K, et al. Upper airway dilating muscle hyperactivity during non-rapid eye movement sleep in English bulldogs. Am Rev Respir Dis 1993;148:185–94.

[12] Veasey SC, Panckeri KA, Hoffman EA, et al. The effects of serotonin antagonists in an animal model of sleep-disordered breathing. Am J Respir Crit Care Med 1996;153:776–86.

[13] Petrof BJ, Hendricks JC, Pack AI. Does upper airway muscle injury trigger a vicious cycle in obstructive sleep apnea? A hypothesis. Sleep 1996;19:465–71.

[14] Petrof BJ, Pack AI, Kelly AM, et al. Pharyngeal myopathy of loaded upper airway in dogs with sleep apnea. J Appl Physiol 1994;76:1746–52.

[15] Holt DE. Laryngeal paralysis. In: King L, editor. Textbook of respiratory disease in dogs and cats. 1st edition. St. Louis (MO): Saunders; 2004. p. 319–28.

[16] Belvisi MG. Overview of the innervation of the lung. Curr Opin Pharmacol 2002;2:211–5.

[17] Canning BJ. Reflex regulation of airway smooth muscle tone. J Appl Physiol 2006;101: 971–85.

[18] McKiernan BC, Johnson LR. Clinical pulmonary function testing in dogs and cats Edition. Vet Clin North Am Small Anim Pract 1992;22:1087–99.

[19] Bedenice D, Rozanski E, Bach J, et al. Canine awake head-out plethysmography (HOP): characterization of external resistive loading and spontaneous laryngeal paralysis. Respir Physiolo Neurobiol 2006;151:61–73.

[20] Miller CJ, McKiernan BC, Pace J, et al. The effects of doxapram hydrochloride (Dopram-V) on laryngeal function in healthy dogs. J Vet Intern Med 2002;16:524–8.

[21] Winters KB, Tidwell AS, Rozanski EA, et al. Characterization of severe small airway disease in a puppy using computed tomography. Vet Radiol Ultrasound 2006;47:470–3.

[22] Lutchen KR, Gillis H. Relationship between heterogeneous changes in airway morphometry and lung resistance and elastance. J Appl Physiol 1997;83:1192–201.

[23] Amis TC, Kurpershoek C. Tidal breathing flow-volume loop analysis for clinical assessment of airway obstruction in conscious dogs. Am J Vet Res 1986;47:1002–6.

[24] Glaab T, Daser A, Braun A, et al. Tidal midexpiratory flow as a measure of airway hyper-responsiveness in allergic mice. Am J Physiol Lung Cell Mol Physiol 2001;280:L565–73.

[25] McKiernan BC, Dye JA, Rozanski EA. Tidal breathing flow-volume loops in healthy and bronchitic cats. J Vet Intern Med 1993;7:388–93.

[26] Zamel N, Kass I, Fleischli GJ. Relative sensitivity of maximal expiratory flow-volume curves using spirometry versus body plethysmograph to detect mild airway obstruction. Am Rev Respir Dis 1973;107:861–3.

[27] Muggenburg BA, Mauderly JL. Cardiopulmonary function of awake, sedated, and anesthe-tized beagle dogs. J Appl Physiol 1974;37:152–7.

[28] Amis TC, Jones HA. Measurement of functional residual capacity and pulmonary carbon monoxide uptake in conscious greyhounds. Am J Vet Res 1984;45:1447–50.

[29] Bedenice D, Bar-Yishay E, Ingenito EP, et al. Evaluation of head-out constant volume body plethysmography for measurement of specific airway resistance in conscious, sedated sheep. Am J Vet Res 2004;65:1259–64.

[30] DuBois A, Botelho S, Comroe JH Jr. A new method for measuring airway resistance in man using a body plethysmograph: values in normal subjects and in patients with respiratory dis-ease. J Clin Invest 1956;35:327–35.

[31] Krell WS, Agrawal KP, Hyatt RE. Quiet-breathing vs. panting methods for determination of specific airway conductance. J Appl Physiol 1984;57:1917–22.

[32] Agrawal KP. Specific airways conductance in guinea pigs: normal values and histamine induced fall. Respir Physiol 1981;43:23–30.

[33] Bach RE, Chan D, Freeman L, et al. Airway dysfunction is associated with higher body con-dition score in healthy Retriever dogs. Am J Vet Res 2007;68(6):670–5.

[34] Nakamura M, Haga T, Sasaki H, et al. Acute effects of cigarette smoke inhalation on periph-eral airways in dogs. J Appl Physiol 1985;58:27–33.

[35] Park SS, Kikkawa Y, Goldring IP, et al. An animal model of cigarette smoking in beagle dogs: correlative evaluation of effects on pulmonary function, defense, and morphology. Am Rev Respir Dis 1977;115:971–9.

Respiratory Defenses in Health and Disease

Leah A. Cohn, DVM, PhD*, Carol R. Reinero, DVM, PhD

Department of Veterinary Medicine and Surgery, University of Missouri-Columbia
College of Veterinary Medicine, 379 East Campus Drive, Clydesdale Hall,
Columbia, MO 65211, USA

OVERVIEW

The challenge presented to the respiratory immune system is to be able to respond to harmful pathogens quickly and effectively yet be able to regulate the resultant inflammatory response tightly to prevent destruction of normal lung tissue. Inhalation continually exposes the airways and air spaces to potentially noxious agents, including particulates, allergens, and microbial organisms; additionally, there is potential for hematogenous delivery of pathogens to the respiratory tract. Therefore, a series of complex and overlapping mechanisms is required to protect the respiratory tract from injury related to these noxious agents. These mechanisms include physical and mechanical defenses, innate immunologic defenses, and specific adaptive immunologic defenses. Adaptive defenses comprise cell-mediated and humoral immune responses. Although these systems provide remarkable protection of the lungs from infection, they are not perfect. Failure of the normal protective mechanisms can lead to potentially life-threatening infection. Further, an exaggerated or misdirected response of these protective mechanisms can lead to immunologically mediated disease states. In fact, the balancing act required for immunologic neutralization of potential pathogens without inappropriate inflammatory amplification may be the greatest challenge faced by pulmonary defense systems [1]. This article reviews the components that collectively provide respiratory defenses and discusses failures of these defenses that allow infection to develop or result in damage to the airways and lungs through an overexuberant response to challenge.

RESPIRATORY DEFENSE MECHANISMS

Physical Defenses

Physical defenses of the respiratory tract include air flow patterns and the anatomic barriers through which air must pass before reaching the lungs; protective reflexes, including cough and sneeze; the epithelial barrier itself; and

---

*Corresponding author. E-mail address: cohnl@missouri.edu (L.A. Cohn).

0195-5616/07/$ – see front matter
doi:10.1016/j.cvsm.2007.05.003

mucociliary clearance mechanisms. The upper respiratory tract removes most inhaled particulates before they ever reach the lungs [2,3]. Turbulent air flow results in impaction of particulates on the mucosal surfaces of the nasal passages and nasopharynx. The scrollwork of the nasal turbinates creates turbulence of air flow and increases the surface area for impaction of particulates. For particles that make it past these initial barriers, the branching pattern of the intrathoracic airways offers an additional opportunity for particulate impaction along mucosal surfaces. Closure of the glottis protects the airways from aspiration during swallowing. Impaction of irritating substances that evade initial barriers can trigger a sneeze reflex (irritation in the nasal passages) or a cough (irritation in the central airways), resulting in expulsion of particulates from the airways.

The mucociliary clearance apparatus promotes routine removal of impacted particulates, including microorganisms [2,4]. The epithelium itself is composed of a variety of cell types, each with distinct functions. The epithelial cells are held together by tight junctions, forming a seal that provides an excellent physical barrier against pathogen entry. In much of the airways, the apical (eg, lumenal) surface of pseudostratified columnar airway epithelium is covered with hair-like projections known as cilia. These cilia beat in a coordinated directional fashion to propel mucus (and the particles trapped within mucus) out of the respiratory tract [4]. The mucosal epithelial surfaces are covered in a bilayered mucus [4]. The outer layer, referred to as the "gel" layer, is a thick viscous material that serves to trap impacted particles and microbes. Just underneath the gel layer is the more serous "sol" layer. It is within the sol layer that epithelial cell cilia beat [4]. Within the sol, cilia bend backward against the direction of mucus flow, essentially into what could be called a "cocked" position (Fig. 1). During this phase of ciliary movement, the gel layer and entrapped particulates remain stationary. Cilia then straighten so that the tips of the cilia contact the bottom of the gel layer; the cilia continue in a craniad motion, pushing the gel and entrapped particulates forward before returning to the cocked position in the sol. Particulates pushed forward in this manner are removed from the respiratory tract by swallowing once they reach the pharynx, or they can be coughed or sneezed out of the airways.

Innate Immunologic Defenses

When physical barriers fail to expel particulates or microbes, innate immunologic responses serve as the next line of defense. Innate defenses require no prior encounter with a potential pathogen to be effective, and they confer no future protection. They are not specific responses to a given pathogen. Innate defenses include compounds secreted from the epithelium and other local cells, complement and inflammatory cascades, and phagocytic and natural killer cells [5–7].

A wide variety of epithelial-derived antimicrobial chemicals form a vitally important part of the innate defense of the respiratory tract. In addition to their barrier function, the respiratory epithelium and submucosal glands produce

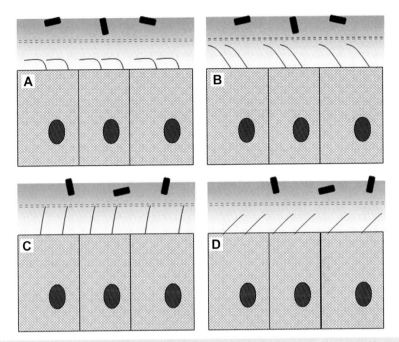

Fig. 1. Lumenal airway epithelium is covered by a mucus bilayer; a thick outer gel layer entraps particulates, whereas the more watery inner sol layer allows for movement of cilia. (A) Within the sol, cilia bend backward against the direction of mucus flow into what could be called a "cocked" position. (B, C) Cilia then straighten so that the tips of the cilia contact the bottom of the gel layer. (D) Cilia continue to move in a craniad direction, pushing the gel and entrapped particulates forward.

and modify airway surface liquid and secrete several chemical defenses. Some of these antimicrobial chemicals, such as defensins, lactoferrin, lysozyme, and cathelicidins, are secreted by phagocytic immune cells and the airway epithelium [5,7–11]. Although these chemicals are released in greater quantity by a single phagocytic cell than by a single epithelial cell, the sheer number of epithelial cells secreting these substances ensures that the epithelial-derived fraction is proportionally greater. The complement system is an enzymatic cascade that functions as a different sort of innate chemical defense [12]. In contrast to the vital role of other chemical defenses, the importance of complement in airway defenses has not been established [10].

The major phagocytic cells of innate defense are the neutrophil and macrophage [12]. These cells bind, ingest, and destroy potential pathogens. Afterward, phagocytic cells or remnants can be transported out of the lung by way of the mucociliary clearance apparatus. In health, few phagocytes (predominantly alveolar macrophages) are found in air spaces. Phagocytes become important when bacteria escape physical barriers and replicate within the lung tissues. Phagocytic binding is triggered by receptor-mediated recognition of pathogens. In the pulmonary vasculature, complement can serve as an opsonin to trigger phagocytosis. Phagocytic cells have receptors capable of recognizing surface molecules displayed by pathogens but not host cells (eg, macrophage mannose receptors, complement receptors, scavenger receptors). Toll-like receptors (TLRs) on phagocytes are prominent among the receptors that recognize molecular patterns common to many potential pathogens [12]. There are many such patterns found on microbes, including components of microbial cell walls, such as lipopolysaccharide from gram-negative bacteria or bacterial genomic DNA containing unmethylated CpG dinucleotides (CpG motifs) [12]. Some of these patterns activate triggers that are more adept at stimulation of phagocytosis and destruction of pathogens, whereas others contribute to the generation of molecules necessary for induction of adaptive immunity, such as cytokines, chemokines, and costimulatory molecules. In addition to phagocytic cells, natural killer cells are involved in innate immunity. Once activated by contact with a target cell, and in concert with locally produced cytokines, killer cells are able to induce programmed cell death (apoptosis) in the target cell [12,13]. Such responses are especially important in target cells infected by intracellular pathogens, including viruses.

The innate immune system is responsible for providing an "immediate" response to the initial encounter with pathogens; however, some pathogens have evolved mechanisms to evade or overwhelm innate immunity. Thus, an additional critical role of the innate immune system is to induce activity of the adaptive immune response by means of interactions between costimulatory molecules on innate immune cells and antigen-specific lymphocytes as well as by producing cytokines and other soluble mediators.

Adaptive Immunologic Defenses

The small concentrations of inhaled pathogens that escape physical and innate defenses are dealt with by adaptive immunologic defenses, as are infectious agents delivered to the lung by a hematogenous route. The adaptive immune response requires several days for maturation, differentiation, and clonal expansion of effector T lymphocytes and plasma cells (antibody-secreting B lymphocytes); however, it is highly specific for pathogens and, importantly, results in immunologic memory (ie, the ability to protect the host more efficiently during future encounters with that specific pathogen) [12]. Adaptive defenses encompass cell-mediated immunity (CMI) and humoral immunity. CMI and humoral immunity use CD4+ T-helper lymphocytes, a cell type that cannot recognize native antigen alone. Instead, antigen must be properly presented to the helper cells by specialized antigen-presenting cells (APCs). Although macrophages often function as APCs in other tissues, the lung relies almost entirely on dendritic cells to present antigen [3,14]. Presentation of the antigen is a key component of the adaptive immune response. When antigen is presented appropriately, CMI or humoral immunity is triggered. CMI is ideally suited to respond to intracellular pathogens, including viral infections; humoral immunity is important in prevention of infection and for resolution of certain established infections. If presentation of antigen is made to the T-helper cells in the absence of appropriate costimulatory signals (including receptor-ligand interactions and chemical cytokine signals), the immune response is aborted and tolerance to the antigen ensues. Induction of tolerance is extremely important at mucosal surfaces that routinely contact the outside world. Were it not for induction of tolerance, even benign particulates (eg, pollens) would induce an immunologic response.

Mucosal-associated lymphoid tissue (MALT) is a distinctive system of lymphoid tissue scattered along body surface sites [12,15]. Specific names are applied to MALT in different areas of the body, including the nasal-associated lymphoid tissue (NALT) and tracheal/bronchial-associated lymphoid tissue (BALT). These tissues are responsible for immune exclusion (noninflammatory surface protection that prevents infection), immune elimination (an evoked response to invaders not repelled by means of exclusion), and even immune regulation (the determination of which antigens should be tolerated and which attacked). MALTs are especially important in performing the inductive aspects of adaptive immunity, meaning that antigens are "sampled" in these tissues and processed in such a way that cell-mediated and humoral effectors can be stimulated. Certain lymphocytes hone in on specific types of MALT by means of cell receptors, circulating between specific mucosal surfaces [15].

Lymphocytes, macrophages, and the cytokines elaborated by each cell type are the key mediators of CMI [12]. When antigen is appropriately presented to T-helper cells by special APCs (eg, dendritic cells), the response is driven toward one of two alternative pathways. Although somewhat of an oversimplification, the T-helper 1 response drives CMI, mononuclear cell activation, and resistance to bacterial and intracellular pathogens [12,13]. The alternative T-helper 2 response promotes IgA and IgE production and is dominant during parasitic infection and in allergic responses [12]. Key effector cells of CMI include CD8+ T-cytotoxic lymphocytes. Unlike T-helper cells, T-cytotoxic cells can recognize antigen presented by most types of nucleated cells. With the help of the CD4+ T cells and in the presence of cellularly derived cytokine signals, T-cytotoxic cells induce apoptotic destruction of infected target cells, and thus destroy the infecting pathogen [12]. CMI is crucial in protection against viral infections and against pulmonary mycobacterial and *Pneumocystis jirovecii* (previously called *Pneumocystis carinii*) infections as well [13].

Humoral immunity depends on immunoglobulins (ie, antibodies) [12]. Immunoglobulins are produced by plasma cells that are derived from B lymphocytes stimulated by antigen (with help from CD4+ lymphocytes). A single plasma cell can produce immunoglobulin that reacts with only one specific antigen; however, the immunoglobulin can be any of several classes, or isotypes. Each isotype has a different structure and function to optimize its performance in a given environment or against a specific group of microbes. Some are especially adept at neutralization of toxins or microbes before they can cause infection, others are extremely efficient at opsonization of microbes or activation of complement, and others are best suited for response to parasitic infections. The isotype of most importance in the upper airways is IgA, whereas IgG and IgM assume greater importance in the pulmonary parenchyma.

IgA protects mucosal surfaces by blocking microbial-epithelial adhesion and uptake, by facilitating mucociliary clearance of agglutinated microbes, and by neutralization of local microbes and toxins [6,12]. Although IgA is produced by plasma cells located just under the epithelial surfaces, it is unique in that it is further processed inside epithelial cells, in which a "secretory component" is added to the dimeric IgA molecule. This component allows IgA to be secreted and maintained on the lumenal mucosal surface, where its protective actions occur.

In the lung parenchyma, monomeric IgG and pentameric IgM serve to protect the host [6]. The smaller IgG is able to reach interstitial lung tissues. Both molecules are effective opsonins that facilitate phagocytic engulfment of microbes and activate the complement cascade. They are less important for immune exclusion of infectious microbes than is IgA but are better capable of dealing with established infection [12].

FAILURE OF RESPIRATORY DEFENSES

Although the respiratory tract possesses myriad defense mechanisms, bacterial, viral, protozoal, or fungal respiratory infections occur on occasion. Viral and fungal pneumonia are most often acquired through inhalation, whereas bacterial pneumonia usually occurs by means of aspiration from the upper airways, by direct extension of infection, or by means of hematogenous infection [16,17]. Many viral and fungal causes of pneumonia are primary pathogens, meaning they possess virulence factors that allow them to cause disease in otherwise healthy animals. Conversely, the pathogens most often responsible for bacterial pneumonia are usually opportunistic pathogens, meaning that they do not cause disease under normal circumstances [18]. Therefore, when bacterial pneumonia does occur, it is important to look for some underlying factor that predisposed the patient to infection.

Abnormalities of systemic or specific respiratory defenses predispose to respiratory infection. When systemic immunodeficiency exists, respiratory infections can occur in conjunction with infections of other body systems. A wide variety of common disease conditions (eg, diabetes mellitus, uremia, retroviral infection in cats) and drug therapies (eg, glucocorticoids, chemotherapeutic drugs) result in systemic immunologic compromise. Congenital immunodeficiency states (eg, severe combined immunodeficiency [SCID], neutrophil function defects, immunoglobulin deficiencies) are less common but cause more severe systemic immunodeficiency, making infections even more likely. Defects in specific respiratory defenses that lead to infection of only the respiratory tract can also be acquired or congenital. Often, defects in respiratory defenses are related to failures of physical or mechanical protective mechanisms.

Failure of Physical Defenses

Significant or sustained breaches in the first and most important barriers to respiratory infection, the physical and mechanical defenses, often lead to infection. For instance, prolonged intubation associated with ventilator therapy bypasses many of the normal physical defenses provided by the upper airways and is often complicated by ventilator-associated pneumonia [19,20]. Animals with laryngeal paralysis, including those that have undergone surgical corrective procedures, have defective laryngeal closure. This breach of a basic mechanical defense leaves them predisposed to aspiration and respiratory infection [21,22]. Animals with profound muscular weakness cannot cough effectively, leaving them more susceptible to bacterial pneumonia.

Injury to the epithelial surfaces of the airway predisposes to secondary bacterial infection. Damage to the nasal turbinates or the overlying mucosal surface from neoplasia, foreign body, or fungal infections often allows the development of secondary bacterial rhinitis. Damage to nasal tissue from feline viral respiratory infections may set the stage for lifelong bouts of recurrent secondary bacterial rhinitis. This might help to explain how cytolytic viruses, such as feline herpesvirus 1, might contribute to idiopathic chronic rhinosinusitis even when active virus cannot be isolated [23]. Airway epithelial damage anywhere along the respiratory tract can set the stage for secondary bacterial infection. Damage might result not only from viral infection but from other types of infection (eg, aspergillosis), inflammation (eg, asthma), inhalation of toxic fumes (eg, smoke), or aspiration of caustic substances (eg, gastric acid).

Even when other physical defenses are intact, defective function of the mucociliary escalator often leads to respiratory infection [4]. This function can be compromised by damaged or denuded airway epithelium, by alterations in the character of the overlying mucus, or by aberrations in ciliary movement. Mucus, secreted by airway epithelium and submucosal glands, is a variable mixture of glycoproteins, low-molecular-weight ions, proteins, lipids, and water. Abnormal mucus composition is postulated to contribute to chronic obstructive pulmonary disease in people [24]; however, no such mucus defects have been investigated in dogs or cats. Although mucolytic drug therapies are sometimes administered to dogs and cats with pneumonia or chronic bronchitis in an attempt to improve mucociliary escalator function, such therapies have not been proven effective. Systemic and airway dehydration might diminish the depth of the mucus sol layer, leading to entrapment of cilia in the gel layer and failure of escalator function [4,25]. Maintenance of airway hydration is critical for the treatment of respiratory infections, including pneumonia. Although not a disease of small animals, one of the major postulated reasons for repeated respiratory infection in people with cystic fibrosis is dehydration of the airway mucus, which results from defective salt and water transport across the airway epithelium [4].

Malfunction of the cilia can result from acquired damage or a congenital defect. Inhaled toxins, such as those found in smoke, are damaging to respiratory cilia, as are oxidants (including those elaborated from inflammatory cells) [26,27]. Cilia can also be damaged by toxins elaborated from infectious agents. In fact, one of the few primary bacterial respiratory pathogens of the dog, *Bordetella bronchiseptica*, is able to infect the airways of healthy hosts because it elaborates a toxin that causes acquired secondary ciliary dyskinesia [28]. *Mycoplasma* spp also paralyze ciliary action.

A syndrome of congenital sinusitis and bronchiectasis was described in people as early as 1904, and the combination of sinusitis, bronchiectasis, and situs inversus (ie, Kartagener's syndrome) was described in 1933 [29,30]. The first functional description of a ciliary defect leading to these syndromes was that of a dynein arm deficiency that caused immotility, resulting in adoption of the name "immotile cilia syndrome" [31]. Since that report by Afzelius [31] in the early 1970s, other acquired defects of cilia resulting in ultrastructural abnormalities or dyskinetic movement have been described. Therefore, the term *primary ciliary dyskinesia* (PCD) is preferred over *immotile cilia syndrome* when describing animals with a congenital ciliary defect.

PCD has been described in many breeds of dogs and occasionally in cats [32–37]. The disorder typically results in recurrent bacterial rhinitis, sinusitis, and pneumonia; initial infections are usually documented before the animal matures [38]. Typically, infections respond to antimicrobial therapy, but repeat infection or relapse occurs after discontinuation of drugs. Because of concomitant ciliary abnormalities in nonrespiratory tissues, hydrocephalus and male infertility are often documented [38]. Because ciliary structures guide embryologic organ placement, situs inversus is present in as many as half of affected patients [32,34]. Physical and clinicopathologic findings in dogs with PCD reflect respiratory infection. Depending on the presence and severity of pneumonia, tachypnea, cyanosis, and pulmonary crackles may be identified. Neutrophilic leukocytosis, potentially with a left shift, is often documented during bouts of pneumonia. Blood gas analysis may indicate hypoxemia and normo- or hypocapnia associated with small airway obstruction. Older dogs may have hyperglobulinemia attributable to recurrent or chronic infection. Radiographic lesions vary with disease severity and chronicity. Lower respiratory disease ranges from mild bronchitis to severe bronchopneumonia with bronchiectasis and lung lobe consolidation.

Diagnosis of PCD is suggested by early and recurrent antimicrobial-responsive respiratory infections, especially in purebred dogs. Although not a sensitive diagnostic method, radiographic documentation of situs inversus is strong supportive evidence of PCD. In sexually mature intact male dogs, examination of sperm motility is likewise a simple and inexpensive supportive diagnostic test. Nuclear scintigraphy can be used as a screening test for the diagnosis of PCD [39]. Anesthesia is induced to allow endotracheal intubation, and a drop of ^{99m}Tc–albumin colloid is placed at the carina. Movement of the droplet is followed and quantified. Although the method cannot definitively differentiate acquired from congenital ciliary dyskinesia, failure of the droplet to move supports the diagnosis of PCD. A nasal mucosal biopsy can yield specimens for evaluation of ciliary movement by means of video-assisted microscopic analysis. This technique requires immediate analysis of fresh tissue using sophisticated technology, and is thus impractical for most clinical cases. Likewise, culture of respiratory epithelium and induction of ciliogenesis is useful but impractical for most veterinary patients [40].

Ultrastructural assessment of cilia requires electron microscopy and is subject to misinterpretation. The sampling procedure, fixation, and examination techniques all have an impact on the results; specimens should only be submitted to laboratories and pathologists with experience and interest in ciliary evaluation. Ultrastructural abnormalities can be seen in some proportion of cilia in animals with no signs of respiratory disease [41]. Misalignment of cilia, microtubular discontinuities, or variations in number or position within the axonemal configuration of cilia can be found secondary to other disease processes [41,42]. Additionally, ultrastructural defects may not be observed in all patients with PCD [42]. Nevertheless, ultrastructural defects are often observed. The most frequently encountered are absence of outer and inner dynein arms; radial spoke defects and transposition defects are also well recognized.

Failure of Innate and Adaptive Immunity

Most failures of innate or adaptive immunity, whether acquired or congenital, lead to infections of multiple body systems rather than to isolated respiratory infection. Repeated infections with opportunistic pathogens should prompt consideration of an immunologic defect. When infections begin early in life, strong consideration should be given to congenital immunodeficiency. Respiratory infections have been described in several dog breeds with congenital immunodeficiency states [43–48]. A thorough discussion of immunodeficiency is beyond the scope of this article, but a limited discussion of immunodeficiency as related to respiratory infection is presented.

Epithelial surfaces rely on secreted IgA to help prevent microbial adherence and infection. IgA deficiency is the most common congenital immunodeficiency of human beings [49] and has been described in several breeds of dogs, including the German Shepherd [50], Shar Pei [51], beagle [52], Irish Wolfhound [53], and Weimaraner [54]. IgA deficiency predisposes to repeated infections of epithelial surfaces, and sinopulmonary infection is the most common manifestation in affected people [49]. Although infections occur, most human beings with IgA deficiency remain healthy. Because immunoglobulins are rarely quantified in healthy animals, we do not know if the same is true for dogs. Complicating our understanding of IgA deficiency in dogs is the fact that low serum or plasma IgA concentrations cannot be equated with deficiencies of functional secreted IgA at mucosal surfaces [55–58]. To investigate IgA deficiency in a young dog with recurrent respiratory infection, secretory IgA should be measured in tears, saliva, or other mucosal secretions [58]. Immunohistochemical staining for IgA-containing B cells in the respiratory mucosa may also be useful [56].

P jirovecii is an opportunistic fungal infection that seldom causes in disease in healthy animals. Pneumonia caused by *Pneumocystis* is well documented in Miniature and Standard Dachshunds and in Cavalier King Charles Spaniels, however [59–65]. Miniature Dachshunds that developed pneumonia caused by *Pneumocystis* at a young age were deficient in several serum immunoglobulin isotypes and demonstrated decreased lymphocyte transformation in response to mitogens, suggesting a combined variable immunodeficiency [60]. Cavalier

King Charles Spaniels tend to develop disease slightly later in life and may have a different sort of immunodeficiency [62]. Although CMI has not been evaluated in infected Cavalier King Charles Spaniels, investigators have speculated that infection may be related to abnormalities in humoral immunity (specifically, IgG) [62]. Unlike most other systemic immunodeficiency syndromes, nonrespiratory infections are seldom documented in dogs with pneumonia caused by *Pneumocystis* [62,66].

Recurrent respiratory infections have been reported in several other poorly characterized but suspected congenital immunodeficiency syndromes. Early-onset rhinitis and bronchopneumonia have been described in more than 24 Irish Wolfhounds from Europe and Canada. Although serum IgA concentrations were lower than expected in many dogs, secreted IgA in bronchoalveolar lavage fluid was increased in some dogs, making IgA deficiency an unlikely explanation for the propensity to development of respiratory infection [53]. Frequent opportunistic respiratory infection has been described in dogs and people with X-linked hypohidrotic ectodermal dysplasia. Thus far, studies have failed to identify a specific immunodeficiency in these dogs [67]. A family of Doberman Pinschers has been described with chronic and recurrent bacterial rhinitis and pneumonia attributable to what was initially believed to be a neutrophil-killing defect [68]. Subsequent evaluation determined that repeated infections were more likely attributable to ciliary dyskinesia rather than to defective neutrophil function [69].

INJURY CAUSED BY RESPIRATORY DEFENSES

The respiratory tract, especially the upper airways, is routinely presented with inhaled particulates. Many are inherently harmless and do not warrant an aggressive response from innate or adaptive immune systems. A complex and incompletely understood system exists in the respiratory tract (as it does in the gastrointestinal tract) to prevent response to harmless antigens. When these systems fail, the inflammatory and immunologic response to otherwise harmless antigens can itself cause disease.

Although inflammation can aid in elimination of infection, tissue injury and loss of function are inherent properties of inflammation. In the airways, these can lead to irritation with increased mucus production, sneeze, cough, or bronchoconstriction. In the lungs, inflammation can lead to impaired gas exchange and respiratory failure. In fact, uncontrolled inflammation or the response to infection underlies some of the most common respiratory disorders, including acute lung injury (ALI) and acute respiratory distress syndrome (ARDS), chronic bronchitis, and asthma [8].

ALI and its more severe progression to ARDS are inflammatory lung disorders characterized by loss of epithelial barrier function, consequent noncardiogenic pulmonary edema, and resultant hypoxia [70,71]. A wide variety of initial insults can lead to the development of ALI or ARDS, including injury of the lung itself or systemic illness accompanied by systemic inflammatory response syndrome. The pathogenesis of ALI or ARDS is complex and incompletely understood. Uncontrolled inflammation in the pulmonary parenchyma, release of chemokines and cytokines, and influx of inflammatory phagocytic cells are key factors [70–73]. Long described as a common and important cause of morbidity and mortality in critically ill people, ALI or ARDS has gained increased attention in small animal patients in recent years [74–78]. In pets even more than in people, this overexuberant pulmonary inflammatory response is associated with extremely high mortality. Interestingly, bacterial pneumonia is a common cause for ALI or ARDS, but ALI or ARDS from any cause (even noninfectious causes like pancreatitis or severe uremia) also increases the likelihood of developing bacterial pneumonia [79].

Feline asthma, characterized by chronic airway inflammation, intermittent reversible airway obstruction, and architectural ("remodeling") changes in the lung, can be induced by a type I hypersensitivity disorder in which normally innocuous inhaled aeroallergens trigger an IgE-mediated inflammatory response [80–82]. The pathogenesis of asthma has been ascribed to T-helper 2 lymphocytes producing cytokines that induce and maintain the allergic inflammatory cascade. Traditionally, feline asthma has been treated with anti-inflammatory corticosteroids (often used in combination with bronchodilator drugs) [81]. Because an inflammatory hypersensitivity reaction is the underlying pathologic defect in asthma, novel therapies seek to inhibit the hypersensitivity or the subsequent inflammatory response [83]. Allergen-specific immunotherapy offers the potential to reverse the asthmatic phenotype, essentially eliminating the disease in the same way it is used to eliminate dermatologic manifestations of atopy [84]. Trials are underway in human beings and cats to evaluate the use of the CpG motif microbial pathogen recognition pattern to "trick" the immune response away from the T-helper 2 phenotype associated with asthma [83,85]. Monoclonal antibodies directed against free IgE are now commercially available for the treatment of asthma in people [86], but these "humanized" monoclonal antibodies cannot be expected to be useful or even safe for the treatment of asthma in cats.

There are many other examples of respiratory disease related to an overexuberant inflammatory response. Atopic rhinitis in human beings is similar to asthma in that it is a type I hypersensitivity [87]. Although common in people, the condition has not been documented clearly in dogs and cats. The cause of chronic bronchitis, a relatively common airway disease of dogs and cats, remains unknown. The disease is characterized by neutrophilic airway inflammation in the absence of airway infection [88,89], however, and thus might represent a disease induced by uncontrolled airway inflammation. Several noninfectious nonneoplastic interstitial lung diseases, including eosinophilic pneumonia, are likely related to an aberrant or exuberant immune or inflammatory response.

SUMMARY

Every breath holds the potential to introduce infectious organisms into the respiratory tract. Despite this continuous exposure, the lungs usually remain sterile. This protection from microbes is attributable, in large measure, to a complex series of physical and mechanical defense mechanisms that exclude pathogens without the need for engagement of an inflammatory or immunologic response to inhaled microbes. Any significant breach in these physical and mechanical defenses can lead to infection. When microbes elude these first lines of defense or when they are presented to the lung through routes other than inhalation, innate immunologic responses are often able to eliminate the potential pathogens. Adaptive cell-mediated and humoral immunologic responses provide for pathogen-specific protection of the respiratory tract and for enhanced protection on future exposure to the same pathogen by means of induction of immunologic memory. Although defects in innate immunity, CMI, and humoral immunity each increase the likelihood of respiratory infection, most of these defects are part of a larger syndrome in which infections of other body systems occur concurrently with respiratory infection. When recurrent infection occurs only in the respiratory tract, physical or mechanical defects are more commonly implicated than systemic immunodeficiency. When an overexuberant immunologic or inflammatory response is triggered within the respiratory tract, the response may cause more profound disease than the threatening agent itself.

References

[1] Crapo JD, Harmsen AG, Sherman MP, et al. Pulmonary immunobiology and inflammation in pulmonary diseases. Am J Respir Crit Care Med 2000;162(5):1983–6.
[2] Chilvers MA, O'Callaghan C. Local mucociliary defense mechanisms. Paediatr Respir Rev 2000;1(1):27–34.
[3] Holt PG. Antigen presentation in the lung. Am J Respir Crit Care Med 2000;162(4 Pt 2): S151–6.
[4] Randell SH, Boucher RC. Effective mucus clearance is essential for respiratory health. Am J Respir Cell Mol Biol 2006;35(1):20–8.
[5] Zaas AK, Schwartz DA. Innate immunity and the lung: defense at the interface between host and environment. Trends Cardiovasc Med 2005;15(6):195–202.
[6] Wilmott RW, Khurana-Hershey G, Stark JM. Current concepts on pulmonary host defense mechanisms in children. Curr Opin Pediatr 2000;12(3):187–93.
[7] Grubor B, Meyerholz DK, Ackermann MR. Collectins and cationic antimicrobial peptides of the respiratory epithelia. Vet Pathol 2006;43(5):595–612.
[8] Whitsett JA. Intrinsic and innate defenses in the lung: intersection of pathways regulating lung morphogenesis, host defense, and repair. J Clin Invest 2002;109(5):565–9.
[9] Whitsett JA. Surfactant proteins in innate host defense of the lung. Biol Neonat 2005;88(3): 175–80.
[10] Hickling TP, Clark H, Malhotra R, et al. Collectins and their role in lung immunity. J Leukoc Biol 2004;75(1):27–33.
[11] McCormack FX. New concepts in collectin-mediated host defense at the air-liquid interface of the lung. Respirology 2006;11(Suppl 1):S7–10.
[12] Tizard IR. Veterinary immunology: an introduction, vol. 1. 7th edition. Philadelphia: Saunders; 2004.
[13] Curtis JL. Cell-mediated adaptive immune defense of the lungs. Proc Am Thorac Soc 2005;2:412–6.
[14] von Garnier C, Filgueira L, Wikstrom M, et al. Anatomical location determines the distribution and function of dendritic cells and other APCs in the respiratory tract. J Immunol 2005;175(3):1609–18.

[15] Xu B, Wagner N, Pham LN, et al. Lymphocyte homing to bronchus-associated lymphoid tissue (BALT) is mediated by L-selectin/PNAd, alpha4beta1 integrin/VCAM-1, and LFA-1 adhesion pathways. J Exp Med 2003;197(10):1255–67.

[16] Mason CM, Nelson S. Normal host defenses and impairments associated with the delayed resolution of pneumonia. Semin Respir Infect 1992;7:243–55.

[17] Macdonald ES, Norris CR, Berghaus RB, et al. Clinicopathologic and radiographic features and etiologic agents in cats with histologically confirmed infectious pneumonia: 39 cases (1991–2000). J Am Vet Med Assoc 2003;223(8):1142–50.

[18] Greene CE, Reinero CN. Bacterial respiratory infections. In: Greene CE, editor. 3rd edition. Infectious diseases of the dog and cat, vol. 1. St. Louis (MO): Saunders Elseivier; 2006. p. 866–82.

[19] Porzecanski I, Bowton DL. Diagnosis and treatment of ventilator-associated pneumonia. Chest 2006;130(2):597–604.

[20] Clare M, Hopper K. Mechanical ventilation: ventilator settings, patient management, and nursing care. Compend Contin Educ Pract Vet 2005;7(4):256–69.

[21] Hammel SP, Hottinger HA, Novo RE. Postoperative results of unilateral arytenoid lateralization for treatment of idiopathic laryngeal paralysis in dogs: 39 cases (1996–2002). J Am Vet Med Assoc 2006;228(8):1215–20.

[22] LaHue TR. Laryngeal paralysis. Semin Vet Med Surg (Sm Anim) 1995;10(2):94–100.

[23] Johnson LR, Foley JE, De Cock HEV, et al. Assessment of infectious organisms associated with chronic rhinosinusitis in cats. J Am Vet Med Assoc 2005;227(4):579–85.

[24] Voynow JA, Gendler SJ, Rose MC. Regulation of mucin genes in chronic inflammatory airway diseases. Am J Respir Cell Mol Biol 2006;34(6):661–5.

[25] Nakagawa NK, Donato-Junior F, Kondo CS, et al. Effects of acute hypovolaemia by furosemide on tracheal transepithelial potential difference and mucus in dogs. Eur Respir J 2004;24(5):805–10.

[26] Jorissen M, Willems T, Van der Schueren B, et al. Secondary ciliary dyskinesia is absent after ciliogenesis in culture. Acta Otorhinolaryngol Belg 2000;54(3):333–42.

[27] Feldman C, Anderson R, Kanthakumar K, et al. Oxidant-mediated ciliary dysfunction in human respiratory epithelium. Free Radic Biol Med 1994;17(1):1–10.

[28] Anderton TL, Maskell DJ, Preston A. Ciliostasis is a key early event during colonization of canine tracheal tissue by Bordetella bronchiseptica. Microbiology 2004;150(Pt 9): 2843–55.

[29] Siewert AW. Über einen Fall von Bronchiectasie bei einem Patienten mit situs inversus viscerum. Berl Klin Wochenschr 1904;41:139–41.

[30] Kartagener M. Zur Pathogenese der Bronchiektasien. Beitr Klin Tuberk 1933;83: 489–501.

[31] Afzelius BA. A human syndrome caused by immotile cilia. Science 1976;193:317–9.

[32] Reichler IM, Hoerauf A, Guscetti F, et al. Primary ciliary dyskinesia with situs inversus totalis, hydrocephalus internus and cardiac malformations in a dog. J Small Anim Pract 2001; 42(7):345–8.

[33] Roperto F, Brunetti A, Saviano L, et al. Morphologic alterations in the cilia of a cat. Vet Pathol 1996;33(4):460–2.

[34] Neil JA, Canapp SO Jr, Cook CR, et al. Kartagener's syndrome in a dachshund dog. J Am Anim Hosp Assoc 2002;38(1):45–9.

[35] Morrison WB, Wilsman NJ, Fox LE, et al. Primary ciliary dyskinesia in the dog. J Vet Intern Med 1987;1(2):67–74.

[36] Maddux JM, Edwards DF, Barnhill MA, et al. Neutrophil function in dogs with congenital ciliary dyskinesia. Vet Pathol 1991;28(5):347–53.

[37] De Scally M, Lobetti RG, Van Wilpe E. Primary ciliary dyskinesia in a Staffordshire bull terrier. J S Afr Vet Assoc 2004;75(3):150–2.

[38] Edwards DF, Patton CS, Kennedy JR. Primary ciliary dyskinesia in the dog. Probl Vet Med 1992;4(2):291–319.

[39] Boeck KD, Proesmans M, Mortelmans L, et al. Mucociliary transport using 99mTc-albumin colloid: a reliable screening test for primary ciliary dyskinesia. Thorax 2005;60:414–7.

[40] Clercx C, Peeters D, Beths T, et al. Use of ciliogenesis in the diagnosis of primary ciliary dyskinesia in a dog. J Am Vet Med Assoc 2000;217(11):1681–5.

[41] Lurie M, Rennert G, Goldenberg S, et al. Ciliary ultrastructure in primary ciliary dyskinesia and other chronic respiratory conditions: the relevance of microtubular abnormalities. Ultrastruct Pathol 1992;16(5):547–53.

[42] Bush A, Cole P, Hariri M, et al. Primary ciliary dyskinesia: diagnosis and standards of care. Eur Respir J 1998;12:982–8.

[43] Lobetti RG. Suspected primary immune deficiency in a Donge de Bordeaux dog. J S Afr Vet Assoc 2002;73(3):133–4.

[44] Couto CG, Krakowka S, Johnson G, et al. In vitro immunologic features of Weimaraner dogs with neutrophil abnormalities and recurrent infections. Vet Immunol Immunopathol 1989;23(1–2):103–12.

[45] McEwan NA, McNeil PE, Thompson H, et al. Diagnostic features, confirmation and disease progression in 28 cases of lethal acrodermatitis of bull terriers. J Small Anim Pract 2000;41(11):501–7.

[46] Jezyk PF, Felsburg PJ, Haskins ME, et al. X-linked severe combined immunodeficiency in the dog. Clin Immunol Immunopathol 1989;52(2):173–89.

[47] Trowald-Wigh G, Ekman S, Hansson K, et al. Clinical, radiological and pathological features of 12 Irish setters with canine leucocyte adhesion deficiency. J Small Anim Pract 2000;41(5):211–7.

[48] Rivas AL, Tintle L, Argentieri D, et al. A primary immunodeficiency syndrome in Shar-Pei dogs. Clin Immunol Immunopathol 1995;74(3):243–51.

[49] Cunningham-Rundles C. Physiology of IgA and IgA deficiency. J Clin Immunol 2001;21(5): 303–9.

[50] Littler RM, Batt RM, Lloyd DH. Total and relative deficiency of gut mucosal IgA in German shepherd dogs demonstrated by faecal analysis. Vet Rec 2006;158(10):334–41.

[51] Moroff SD, Hurvitz AI, Peterson ME, et al. IgA deficiency in shar-pei dogs. Vet Immunol Immunopathol 1986;13(3):181–8.

[52] Glickman LT, Shofer FS, Payton AJ, et al. Survey of serum IgA, IgG, and IgM concentrations in a large beagle population in which IgA deficiency had been identified. Am J Vet Res 1988;49(8):1240–5.

[53] Clercx C, Reichler I, Peeters D, et al. Rhinitis/bronchopneumonia syndrome in Irish Wolfhounds. Journal of Veterinary Internal Medicine 2003;17(6):843–9.

[54] Foale RD, Herrtage ME, Day MJ. Retrospective study of 25 young weimaraners with low serum immunoglobulin concentrations and inflammatory disease. Vet Rec 2003;153(18): 553–8.

[55] Ginel PJ, Novales M, Lozano MD, et al. Local secretory IgA in dogs with low systemic IgA levels. Vet Rec 1993;132(13):321–3.

[56] Norris CR, Gershwin LJ. Evaluation of systemic and secretory IgA concentrations and immunohistochemical stains for IgA-containing B cells in mucosal tissues of an Irish setter with selective IgA deficiency. J Am Anim Hosp Assoc 2003;39(3):247–50.

[57] Peters IR, Calvert EL, Hall EJ, et al. Measurement of immunoglobulin concentrations in the feces of healthy dogs. Clin Diagn Lab Immunol 2004;11(5):841–8.

[58] German AJ, Hall EJ, Day MJ. Measurement of IgG, IgM and IgA concentrations in canine serum, saliva, tears and bile. Vet Immunol Immunopathol 1998;64(2):107–21.

[59] Lobetti RG, Leisewitz AL, Spencer JA. Pneumocystis carinii in the miniature dachshund: case report and literature review. J Small Anim Pract 1996;37(6):280–5.

[60] Lobetti R. Common variable immunodeficiency in miniature dachshunds affected with Pneumocystis carinii pneumonia. J Vet Diagn Invest 2000;12(1):39–45.

[61] Botha WS, van Rensburg I. Pneumocystosis: a chronic respiratory distress syndrome in the dog. J S Afr Vet Assoc 1979;50:173–9.

[62] Watson PJ, Wotton P, Eastwood J, et al. Immunoglobulin deficiency in Pneumocystis pneumonia. J Vet Intern Med 2006;20(3):523–7.

[63] Canfield PJ, Church DB, Malik R. Pneumocystis pneumonia in a dog. Australian Veterinary Practitioner 1993;23(3):150–4.

[64] Hagiwara Y, Fujiwara S, Takai H, et al. Pneumocystis carinii pneumonia in a cavalier king charles spaniel. J Vet Med Sci 2001;63(3):349–51.

[65] Ramsey IK, Foster A, McKay J, et al. Pneumocystis carinii pneumonia in two cavalier king charles spaniels. Vet Rec 1997;140(14):372–3.

[66] Furuta T, Nogami S, Kojima S, et al. Spontaneous Pneumocystis carinii infection in the dog with naturally acquired generalised demodicosis. Vet Rec 1994;134(16):423–4.

[67] Casal ML, Mauldin EA, Ryan S, et al. Frequent respiratory tract infections in the canine model of X-linked ectodermal dysplasia are not caused by an immune deficiency. Vet Immunol Immunopathol 2005;107(1–2):95–104.

[68] Breitschwerdt EB, Brown TT, De Buysscher EV, et al. Rhinitis, pneumonia, and defective neutrophil function in the Doberman pinscher. Am J Vet Res 1987;48(7):1054–62.

[69] Cohn LA. Evaluation of doberman pinscher dogs related to a family of dogs with respiratory disease [PhD dissertation]. Raleigh (NC): Veterinary Medical Sciences, North Carolina State University; 1994.

[70] Matthay MA, Zimmerman GA. Acute lung injury and the acute respiratory distress syndrome: four decades of inquiry into pathogenesis and rational management. Am J Respir Cell Mol Biol 2005;33(4):319–27.

[71] Ware L, Matthay M. The acute respiratory distress syndrome. N Engl J Med 2000;342:1344–9.

[72] Puneet P, Moochhala S, Bhatia M. Chemokines in acute respiratory distress syndrome. Am J Physiol Lung Cell Mol Physiol 2005;288(1):L3–15.

[73] Mukhopadhyay S, Hoidal JR, Mukherjee TK. Role of TNF alpha in pulmonary pathophysiology. Respir Res 2006;7:125.

[74] Jarvinen AK, Saario E, Andresen E, et al. Lung injury leading to respiratory distress syndrome in young dalmatian dogs. J Vet Intern Med 1995;9(3):162–8.

[75] Walker T, Tidwell AS, Rozanski EA, et al. Imaging diagnosis: acute lung injury following massive bee envenomation in a dog. Vet Radiol Ultrasound 2005;46(4):300–3.

[76] Parent C, King L, Walker L, et al. Clinical and clinicopathologic finding in dogs with acute respiratory distress syndrome: 19 cases (1985–1993). J Am Vet Med Assoc 1996;208:1419–27.

[77] Lopez A, Lane I, Hanna P. Adult respiratory distress syndrome in a dog with necrotizing pancreatitis. Can Vet J 1995;36:240–1.

[78] DeClue AE, Cohn LA. Acute respiratory distress syndrome in dogs and cats: a review of clinical findings and pathophysiology. J Vet Em Crit Care, in press.

[79] Dreyfuss D, Ricard JD. Acute lung injury and bacterial infection. Clin Chest Med 2005;26(1):105–12.

[80] Byers GG, Dhupa N. Feline bronchial asthma: pathophysiology and diagnosis. Compend Contin Educ Pract Vet 2005;27(6):418–25.

[81] Padrid P. Feline asthma. Diagnosis and treatment. Vet Clin North Am Small Anim Pract 2000;30(6):1279–93.

[82] Norris Reinero C, Decile KC, Berghaus RD, et al. An experimental model of allergic asthma in cats sensitized to house dust mite or bermuda grass allergen. Int Arch Allergy Immunol 2004;135:117–31.

[83] Leath TM, Singla M, Peters SP. Novel and emerging therapies for asthma. Drug Discov Today 2005;10(23–24):1647–55.

[84] Reinero CR, Byerly JR, Berghaus RD, et al. Rush immunotherapy in an experimental model of feline allergic asthma. Vet Immunol Immunopathol 2006;110(1–2):141–53.

[85] Reinero CR, Byerly JR, Berghaus LJ, et al. Dissociation between airway inflammation and clinical signs of bronchoconstriction with CpG motifs in experimental feline asthma. J Vet Intern Med 2005;19(3):405A.

[86] Strunk RC, Bloomberg GR. Omalizumab for asthma. N Engl J Med 2006;354(25): 2689–95.

[87] Powe DG, Jagger C, Kleinjan A, et al. 'Entopy': localized mucosal allergic disease in the absence of systemic responses for atopy. Clin Exp Allergy 2003;33(10):1374–9.

[88] Nikula KJ, Green FH. Animal models of chronic bronchitis and their relevance to studies of particle-induced disease. Inhal Toxicol 2000;12(Suppl 4):123–53.

[89] McKiernan BC. Diagnosis and treatment of canine chronic bronchitis. Twenty years of experience. Vet Clin North Am Small Anim Pract 2000;30(6):1267–78.

Approach to the Respiratory Patient

Carrie J. Miller, DVM

Wheat Ridge Veterinary Specialists, 3695 Kipling Street, Wheat Ridge, CO 80033, USA

Several challenges arise when evaluating a dog or cat with respiratory disease. Most of the respiratory tract is encompassed within bony structures, making palpation and visual assessment difficult. The respiratory system also has a high degree of ventilatory reserve and some regenerative capability as well [1,2]. This can make respiratory diseases difficult to appreciate clinically until the disease is fairly severe. Additionally, diseases primarily affecting other organs can result in respiratory embarrassment even if the respiratory system is healthy. The history of patients with respiratory disease can be ambiguous, because some owners can have a difficult time in recognizing or describing respiratory abnormalities [3]. These are all challenges that a clinician faces when evaluating a patient with respiratory disease. There are some non-invasive diagnostics that aid in the diagnosis of respiratory disease; however, other more invasive tests can require anesthesia, which represents a potential hazard with a respiratory patient. This article focuses on reviewing the function of the respiratory system and how best to identify and diagnose cats and dogs with respiratory disease by implementing a thorough history and physical examination as well as appropriate diagnostic testing.

FUNCTIONAL ANATOMY OF THE RESPIRATORY TRACT

The anatomy of the respiratory tract is composed of a series of air passages with the primary goal of oxygen (O_2) delivery and carbon dioxide (CO_2) exchange at the level of the pulmonary capillaries. The respiratory tract begins at the nasal cavity, where the main functions are to humidify, filter, and warm inspired air. Particles greater than 20 µm are filtered within the nasal turbinates [4]. The lateral nasal glands also can aid in heat dissipation and thermoregulation in the dog [5,6]. The nasal cavity ends and the pharynx begins at the level of the choana, and it extends just rostral to the larynx at the intrapharyngeal ostium. The pharynx represents a defined area rather than an organized structure with obvious boundaries. It is considered part of the respiratory system as well as part of the gastrointestinal system. The overlapping function of the pharynx demonstrates why aspiration pneumonia is a relatively common occurrence [7].

E-mail address: cmiller@wrah.com

0195-5616/07/$ – see front matter
doi:10.1016/j.cvsm.2007.05.014

The larynx is a complex musculocartilaginous structure that provides the primary protection for the trachea and lower airways from aspiration of food, water, secretions, or other debris. The rostral boundaries of the larynx are defined by the arytenoid cartilages and vocal folds (dorsal and lateral) and the epiglottis (ventral). The caudal boundaries are defined by the thyroid and cricoid cartilages. The area between the paired arytenoid cartilages is termed the *rima glottis*. The rima glottis is protected by folding over of the epiglottis and by adduction of the arytenoid cartilages during swallowing [7,8]. The larynx also functions in vocalization of cats and dogs. These respiratory structures (nasal cavity, pharynx, and larynx) are termed the *upper airways* [9].

The larynx is connected to the trachea, a noncollapsible, cartilaginous, tube-like structure that extends to the lungs. The lower airways begin at the level of the trachea [9]. The trachea is a series of C-shaped rigid cartilage rings. The dorsal aspect of these rings is bridged by the transversely oriented trachealis muscle. These rings are connected to each other by longitudinally oriented annular ligaments. The trachea serves mainly to conduct air to the lower airways by means of a low-resistance system [7]. The mucociliary tree of the tracheal epithelium consists of microscopic cilia that beat in the orad direction to aid in removing secretions and debris from the lower airways. The sensory nerves lining the tracheal and laryngeal epithelium aid in eliciting the cough reflex. None of the structures discussed here directly participate in gas exchange, with their primary roles including filtering and warming of air and protection of the more distal airways [10].

The trachea ends at the carina, where it branches into the right and left mainstem bronchi. These bronchi then branch into lobar bronchi. On the left side of the thorax, the lobar bronchi include the left cranial lung lobe (cranial and caudal aspects) and the left caudal lung lobe. On the right side, the principal bronchus gives rise to the right cranial lung lobe, the right middle lung lobe, the accessory lung lobe, and the right caudal lung lobe. Each lobar bronchus branches into segmental bronchi, which then undergo dichotomous branching to form the smaller bronchioles. Bronchioles give rise to alveolar ducts, alveolar sacs, and alveoli [7,10]. Gas exchange occurs at the level of the respiratory bronchioles, alveolar ducts, alveolar sacs, and alveoli [11].

O_2 and CO_2 are exchanged by means of passive diffusion generated by a pressure gradient. Gases must pass through the respiratory barrier composed of the alveolar epithelium, alveolar interstitium, and capillary endothelium. Conditions that lead to hypoxemia include (1) low inspired oxygen fraction (FIO_2), (2) hypoventilation, (3) thickening of the respiratory barrier, (4) shunting of pulmonary blood, and (5) physiologic dead space [12,13]. Shunting of pulmonary blood and physiologic dead space can be described as ventilation-perfusion inequality. Shunting of pulmonary blood occurs when there is not enough ventilation to oxygenate fully the blood flowing through the alveolar capillaries (ie, atelectatic lung, alveolar edema). Physiologic dead space occurs when ventilation of alveoli is normal but the alveolar blood flow is low, causing insufficient oxygenation of the alveolar blood (ie, pulmonary thromboembolus

[PTE], congenital cardiac shunts). A two- to threefold increase in the thickness of the respiratory barrier impairs O_2 diffusion [11]. This can occur with edema within the alveolar interstitium or fibrosis of the interstitium, although clinical signs are not apparent until disease is severe.

Most of the O_2 in blood is carried bound to hemoglobin, and only 3% of the O_2 is in the dissolved state. CO_2 is carried by several different chemical forms, including, HCO_3 (70%), CO_2 (7%), and CO_2 bound to hemoglobin (23%). Through diffusion of CO_2 out of the respiratory tract, the lungs also play an important role in acid-base regulation [11,13]. An in-depth discussion of acid-base regulation is beyond the scope of this article, and the reader is referred to a multitude of excellent sources for a detailed discussion of acid-base respiratory physiology [11,14].

HISTORICAL FINDINGS

It is imperative that animals in respiratory distress be stabilized before time is taken to obtain a thorough history. Stabilization may include O_2 therapy, appropriate medications (ie, sedatives, bronchodilators, glucocorticoids, diuretics), and then a brief history. Once the patient is stabilized, a thorough history is crucial, because some respiratory patients can have a medical history that spans months to years. Other body systems can have marked effects on the respiratory system; thus, the history should also include questions regarding the patient's overall health. Most patients with respiratory disease present with a primary complaint of sneezing, nasal discharge, reverse sneezing, coughing, epistaxis, labored breathing, or exercise intolerance. Other less common complaints include syncope, regurgitation, dysphagia, dysphonia, collapse, or cachexia [3,15]. Because many fungal and parasitic diseases initially infect the respiratory system, a travel history is particularly relevant. Certain questions targeted at the respiratory system can help to narrow the list of differential diagnoses.

If labored breathing is a primary complaint, the owners should be asked to expand on this description. Some owners perceive panting or reverse sneezing as a form of labored breathing, and this can be misleading to the clinician. The clinician should discuss with the owner whether the patient's chest wall is actually moving more than normal and if the patient is tiring more than usual. A healthy cat or dog with normal respiratory effort has minimal movement of the chest wall during respiration at rest [16]. It is also important to determine when the labored breathing is noticed. Patients that experience more labored breathing with heat or excitement classically have diseases affecting the upper airways (eg, brachycephalic syndrome, laryngeal paralysis).

Many owner complaints focus on noisy breathing or a change in the bark or meow (dysphonia). The owner should describe the type of abnormal sound appreciated. A high-pitched raspy noise helps to describe stridor, whereas a gurgly low-pitched sound can describe snoring (stertor). Changes in voice suggest diseases of the upper airways, particularly laryngeal and pharyngeal diseases [3,7].

Some owners may complain of concurrent vomiting or regurgitation. The clinician should inquire whether the animal is coughing and then regurgitating (posttussive wretch) or whether it is truly vomiting. Some brachycephalic dogs may have a history of regurgitation or vomiting because of chronic respiratory disease [17,18]. The owner should also be asked to describe the nature, frequency, and circumstances of occurrence of a cough, if present. Laryngeal and tracheal diseases tend to cause a dry nonproductive cough, whereas airway or parenchymal diseases can produce a wet cough with a significant amount of secretions [3,7].

Because the respiratory system has a high ventilatory reserve, respiratory diseases may exist for much longer than is apparent to the owner or veterinarian. Some owners consider their pet's behavior as normal because it has been going on for so long. A bulldog that snores at night or a Yorkshire Terrier that coughs when excited, for example, may be interpreted as normal by the owner. Taking the time to ask specific questions about the respiratory history of the dog or cat can aid the clinician in determining the most likely disease responsible for clinical signs.

PHYSICAL EXAMINATION

The physical examination is extremely important in assessing respiratory health. Much can be learned simply by watching the animal breathe; certain abnormal breathing patterns can often aid in locating the anatomic position and nature of the disease. Even before approaching the animal, an attempt should be made to observe the animal while talking to the owner. This allows the clinician to appreciate any abnormalities that the owner is describing [7,19]. A dog or cat breathing at rest shows minimal movement of the chest wall. When the breathing becomes more labored, the ribs are pulled caudally and laterally by the diaphragm and chest wall muscles and the abdomen moves slightly outward. Labored breathing may be accompanied by recruitment of additional accessory chest wall muscles as well as nasal and pharyngeal dilator muscles. Flaring of the nostrils or contraction of the abdominal muscles indicates severe labored breathing [16].

Certain breathing patterns can be associated with disease at a specific location in the respiratory tract. Short shallow respirations with small tidal volumes are suggestive of stiff noncompliant lungs or restricted expansion of the lungs from pleural or thoracic wall diseases. Prolonged deep inspirations tend to be associated with laryngeal, pharyngeal, or cervical tracheal diseases, whereas prolonged inspiration and expiration are more compatible with a fixed obstruction. Because of the dynamic nature of respiration, narrowing of small airways has a much more profound effect on expiration than inspiration. Clinically, this appears as an expiratory or abdominal push. Some dogs may have hypertrophy of the abdominal muscles secondary to long-standing small airway disease. By watching and gaining experience in how the animal breathes, a clinician can already have narrowed the list of differential diagnoses before any diagnostics are performed. Orthopnea is defined as difficulty in breathing, except in an erect sitting or standing position. This is usually present in animals with severe respiratory distress [7,16].

Once observations have been made regarding the patient's respiratory rate, effort, pattern, and posture, the clinician should perform a complete physical examination of the entire respiratory system. Initially, the mucous membranes should be checked for any indication of cyanosis or pallor, which would indicate the need for immediate O_2 supplementation. Cyanosis becomes clinically apparent when the deoxygenated hemoglobin concentration reaches 5 g/dL and indicates that the patient is in true respiratory distress [20]. Both nares should be checked for air flow. This can be accomplished in several different manners. Suggestions include listening for air flow through the nares with a stethoscope, placing a frozen glass slide in front of the nares and watching for condensation, or placing the examiner's ear next to the animal's nares to listen for normal air flow. Facial symmetry should be noted as well. The patient's mouth should be opened to evaluate for any hard or soft palate abnormalities as well as to evaluate the upper dental arcade for evidence of oronasal fistulas or tooth abscessation. Some patients may allow the clinician to get a brief look at the larynx, but this should not be considered a sufficient evaluation of the laryngeal and pharyngeal area. Note any excessive reverse sneezing, which could indicate inflammation or irritation to the nasopharynx [7,21,22].

The cervical trachea should be digitally palpated. Abnormalities that might be encountered include an easily compressible trachea, a hypoplastic trachea, or a cervical mass that may be compressing the trachea. Tracheal sensitivity can be evaluated by applying mild to moderate digital compression of the cervical trachea. When a cough is easily elicited (increased tracheal sensitivity), generalized airway inflammation or irritation should be presumed. If a cough is elicited with tracheal palpation, the clinician should note whether the cough is dry or wet in nature, because most parenchymal diseases produce secretions and a wet cough [3,7].

Physical examination of the pulmonary parenchyma is more limited than that of other areas of the respiratory tract, given that it is completely encompassed within the thoracic cavity. The thoracic cavity should be palpated for any defects or masses that could be affecting the respiratory system. The clinician's only tools to evaluate the lower airways on the physical examination are by observing the rate, pattern, and nature of the animal's breathing as well as lung auscultation. Lung auscultation was first introduced by Laennec in 1819 as a way of describing the explosive and musical sounds heard within the lungs when listening with a stethoscope. Until the 1950s, lung sound terminology was confusing and unclear. It included such terms as rales (moist, mucous, sonorous, sibilant, and crackling), rhonchi (dry and wet), and wheezes to describe adventitious lung sounds. These definitions became more unclear with time, which led to the proposal by Robertson and Coope in 1957 to divide adventitious lung sounds into two new and simple groups. These two new groups include continuous sounds (wheezes) and intermittent sounds (crackles). Wheezes are defined as musical sounds that are primarily classified according to pitch (high and low) and timing (inspiratory and expiratory) [23]. Wheezes are thought to be generated primarily by airway narrowing, stenosis, or obstruction. Crackles are defined as short, explosive, nonmusical sounds and are primarily defined by pitch (high and low) and timing (inspiratory and expiratory). Crackles are typically produced by a delayed opening of small airways attributable to an abnormal fluid-air interface (ie, pneumonia, pulmonary edema, bronchitis) (Table 1). Normal breath sounds in the dog and cat include soft low-pitched airway sounds that are generally only appreciated on inspiration. In some cats, it may be difficult to appreciate normal inspiratory breath sounds [3]. When these sounds become loud or prominent on expiration, the descriptive term used most frequently is increased breath sounds or increased bronchovesicular sounds. Sounds generated in the upper airways can often be auscultated within the lungs (referred airway sounds). These can be differentiated from true lung sounds by auscultating over the cervical trachea and larynx and determining where the sound is the loudest. The sound is generated from the spot where it is the loudest [7,19,22].

Stridor is used to describe upper airway noise. It is described as a harsh high-pitched respiratory sound and is often associated with laryngeal obstruction. Stertor is defined as snoring or sonorous breathing and is often associated with pharyngeal or nasopharyngeal disease. Because these are both sounds associated with the upper airways, they are often easy to detect during physical examination. Occasionally, these sounds can only be appreciated with auscultation over the larynx and cervical trachea [3,7,12,24]. Although auscultation is a useful tool, the sensitivity and specificity are largely understudied in veterinary medicine. One study demonstrated good correlation between abnormal adventitious sounds and thoracic trauma; however, other studies are lacking

Table 1
Classification of respiratory sounds in small animal veterinary medicine

Description	Definition
Breath sounds	These are the normal, faint, low-pitched sounds heard through the chest wall of a healthy patient
	These sounds are louder on inspiration and are sometimes barely perceptible in cats
Crackles	Short, explosive, nonmusical sounds primarily defined by pitch (high and low) and timing (inspiration versus expiration)
Wheezes	Musical sounds primarily described by pitch (high and low) and timing (inspiration versus expiration)
Stridor	Harsh high-pitched respiratory sound, often associated with laryngeal obstruction
Stertor	Act of snoring or sonorous breathing, often associated with pharyngeal or nasopharyngeal disease

Data from Corcoran B. Clinical evaluation of the patient with respiratory disease. In: Ettinger SJ, Feldman EC, editors. Textbook of veterinary internal medicine. 5th edition. Philadelphia: WB Saunders; 2000. p. 1035; and Forgacs P. Terminology. In: Lung sounds. London: Baillere Tindall; 1978. p. 1–6.

[25]. Even with normal lung sounds, diagnostics should be pursued if there is historical or physical evidence to suggest respiratory embarrassment.

DIAGNOSTIC TESTING

Many diagnostic aids are available to the clinician to help identify and describe the type of respiratory disease present. Some of these tests also help in quantifying the degree of respiratory disease present. It is imperative with respiratory patients that the potential hazard of any test be considered, because minor stress can lead to decompensation of these patients [12].

Hematology, Biochemistry, and Serology

Patients that have a respiratory disease often have hematology and biochemical profiles that are unremarkable or show nonspecific changes. The most important contribution of hematology and biochemistry profiles is to uncover any systemic or metabolic diseases that might be affecting the respiratory system (ie, acid-base imbalance, anemia). Some relatively common hematology findings associated with respiratory disease include polycythemia from chronic hypoxia, leukocytosis with respiratory infections, or eosinophilia with pulmonary infiltrates with eosinophils (PIE) or parasitic lung infections. Basophilia can also be suggestive of heartworm infection [3]. Eosinophilia can be seen in cats with bronchial disease; however, there is no absolute association with disease [26]. Cats with respiratory distress and eosinophilia should not be presumed to have feline asthma or bronchopulmonary disease. Whenever hemoptysis or unexplained respiratory distress is present, a coagulation profile should be performed to rule out warfarin toxicity [3,27]. Serology can be beneficial in the diagnosis of pulmonary mycotic diseases, particularly coccidioidomycosis or cryptococcosis. In cats, serology for feline leukemia virus (FeLV) and feline immunodeficiency virus (FIV) can aid in ruling out any underlying immune deficiency [3,28].

Radiography

Thoracic radiography is an invaluable tool for investigating respiratory disease. Even so, diagnostic information may be limited by poor radiographic technique, poor patient cooperation, and an inherently low diagnostic sensitivity and specificity. The reader is referred to several excellent veterinary resources that explain the details of thoracic radiographic technique [29,30]. Three views of the thorax are often recommended to maximize lesion detection and to minimize superimposition of thoracic structures. The importance of sedation or general anesthesia should be emphasized as a tool to aid in proper patient positioning. Patient rotation may cause normal thoracic structures to appear abnormal or may hide abnormalities within the thorax because of superimposition of other structures. Always keep in mind that thoracic radiology does have low specificity and that it is rare to form a definitive diagnosis from thoracic radiographs alone. Thoracic radiography, however, is useful in leading to a working list of potential differential diagnoses. Specific radiographic signs can suggest certain diseases and narrow the list of differential diagnoses [29].

The assessment of any radiograph should follow a set procedure and should be consistent for the reader. This ensures that subtle radiographic changes are not overlooked and prevents misdiagnosis caused by not reading the entire radiograph. Most clinicians find it beneficial to evaluate the structures outside the pulmonary parenchyma first to prevent inadvertently focusing only on the pulmonary system. All bony structures should be evaluated for abnormalities, including lysis, proliferation, osteoporosis, or fractures. The diaphragm and mediastinum should also be checked for anatomic abnormalities. The position and size of the cardiac silhouette, great vessels, and associated structures should be assessed, and the radiograph should be reviewed for sternal or hilar lymphadenopathy [29].

The trachea should then be evaluated for narrowing, compression, or deviations in the cervical and intrathoracic region. An undulating or deviating trachea can be a normal variant or a result of improper patient positioning. Elevation of the trachea at the level of the carina can indicate a mediastinal or cardiac mass [31]. Occasionally, static radiographs can detect changes in the luminal diameter of the mainstem bronchi.

Within the pulmonary parenchyma, pulmonary vessels can be visualized and the airways are seen between the paired artery and vein. Bronchial walls are not normally visible, except in the central area or if they are calcified (an age-related change). If the walls become thickened because of inflammation, end-on ring structures (doughnuts) or parallel line markings (tramlines or train tracks) can be visualized. These findings are thought to reflect pathologic change. An interstitial pattern can be described as linear densities that give a hazy appearance to the lung field and obscure visualization of the vasculature. This pattern can be difficult to discern and is highly sensitive to obesity or changes in radiographic technique. An alveolar pattern appears as a soft tissue density in the lung containing air bronchograms, airways outlined by infiltrated pulmonary parenchyma (Fig. 1). These appear as air-filled structures (often branching) against the soft tissue opacity of the lung. An alveolar pattern without the presence of air bronchograms can occur with pulmonary masses, atelectasis, lung lobe torsion, or pulmonary granuloma. The patterns described are generalizations, and several different patterns or a spectrum of the patterns can often be found on thoracic radiographs [29,32]. These patterns describe where the pathologic change is located (bronchioles, interstitium, or alveoli) but do not provide a definitive diagnosis.

CT/Thoracic Ultrasound/Fluoroscopy

Many of the previous uses for fluoroscopy in small animal medicine are presently being replaced by the use of CT and thoracic ultrasound. Fluoroscopy is still used in some specialty private practices and academic institutions to detect tracheal or airway collapse. The dynamic nature of fluoroscopy makes it much more sensitive and specific for tracheal collapse than thoracic radiographs. The extent of the trachea involved can be accurately assessed as well as the dynamic change in the tracheal diameter [29].

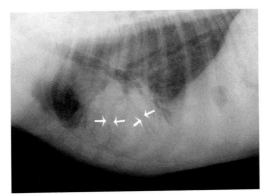

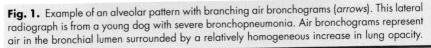

Fig. 1. Example of an alveolar pattern with branching air bronchograms (*arrows*). This lateral radiograph is from a young dog with severe bronchopneumonia. Air bronchograms represent air in the bronchial lumen surrounded by a relatively homogeneous increase in lung opacity.

Thoracic ultrasound has emerged as a relatively new tool in thoracic imaging. Thoracic ultrasound is best used if preceded by thoracic radiographs so as to define the location of the lesion. Structures within the lungs that are surrounded by aerated lung are not accessible with thoracic ultrasound. The modality is most useful when evaluating cardiac or mediastinal masses (the ventral portion of the mediastinum), consolidated or collapsed lung lobes, pleural effusion, or thoracic wall masses or when looking for diaphragmatic hernias. If the lesion can be visualized, a fine-needle aspirate or biopsy can be attempted with sedation or general anesthesia, depending on the ultrasonographer's comfort level with the appearance of the mass [29,33].

The introduction of thoracic CT in veterinary medicine has allowed subtle changes within the thoracic cavity to be more easily detected and described. This is attributable to CT's inherent superiority in contrast resolution as compared with radiography [34]. It is also used commonly for planning radiation therapy for nasal neoplasia. CT can also be valuable when thoracic radiographs are normal, although lung pathologic change is still suspected. CT angiography is being introduced in veterinary medicine to detect PTE [35]. In experimentally induced PTEs in dogs, the PTE was detected in 64% to 76% of the dogs, although detection depends highly on user experience. In human patients, CT angiography has replaced ventilation:perfusion (V/Q) scintigraphy as the diagnostic tool used with PTEs [29]. CT has also been used with variable results in dogs with spontaneous pneumothorax, in which the underlying lung lesion can be difficult to see at the time of exploratory thoracotomy [36]. For a more complete description of the role of CT in respiratory disease, see the article by Johnson elsewhere in this issue.

Rhinoscopy and Bronchoscopy

Endoscopy is the best tool to visualize the entirety of the respiratory tract. In addition to direct visualization, endoscopy (rhinoscopy and bronchoscopy) allows for collection of tissue and fluid samples and removal of foreign bodies. Initially, the caudal nasal chamber and nasopharynx are visualized using a flexible fiberoptic endoscope or videoendoscope (5-mm bronchoscope or 7.9-mm gastroscope is most common) (Fig. 2). A multipurpose, rigid, 2.7-mm telescope is most useful when evaluating the rostral nares. This allows visualization of the dorsal, middle, and ventral meatuses and assessment of turbinate quantity and health [37–39]. When significant turbinate destruction is present, the frontal sinuses may also be visualized. Biopsies are most easily obtained when visualization is achieved with the rigid scope. Rhinoscopy and nasal biopsy can cause significant epistaxis, and the patient should be monitored for several hours at least before leaving the hospital.

Bronchoscopy in small animal patients is performed in sternal recumbency to minimize lung atelectasis and subsequent hypoxia. Bronchoscopy is most commonly performed with a 5.0-mm flexible fiberoptic bronchoscope or videoendoscope, although a 2.5-mm scope may be preferable in cats to limit obstruction of exhaled air. Bronchoscopy should begin by first evaluating the larynx (see section on laryngoscopy). The scope is then passed into the proximal trachea, with the endoscopist making sure not to contaminate the scope with the oral bacterial flora. The normal tracheobronchial mucosa has a light pink color, and mucosal vessels are readily visible (Fig. 3). Edema causes blanching of the mucosa and obscure visualization of the vessels. The trachea should be evaluated for the presence of mucus, hyperemia, or dynamic collapse. In some cases of chronic airway inflammation, nodules can be seen along the more distal tracheal and bronchial mucosa, indicating the chronicity of disease. Beyond the level of the carina, the endoscopist should be aware of the appropriate orientation of all lobar bronchi to determine the precise location within the bronchial tree. Airway anatomic nomenclature has been well described for the dog and aids in describing the location of specific lesions [40]. This aids in describing the location of any abnormalities found during bronchoscopy.

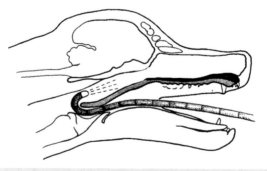

Fig. 2. Schematic representation of retrograde rhinoscopy using a flexible fiberoptic endoscope to examine the nasopharynx of a dog. (*Adapted from* Pook HA, Meric SM. Caudal nasal cyst in a dog: retrograde rhinoscopic management. J Am Anim Hosp Assoc 1990;26(2):170; with permission.)

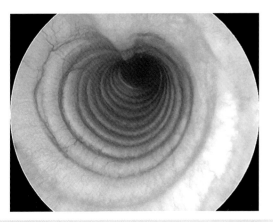

Fig. 3. Appearance of a normal canine trachea during tracheoscopy. There should be minimal secretions within the trachea. The tracheal mucosa appears light pink, with the capillary blood vessels easily visualized.

Fig. 4 demonstrates the positioning of the right and left mainstem bronchi as well as the location of the lobar bronchi. The amount of secretions, mucosa color, and dynamic collapse of any airways should be noted at this level as well. Widening of the carina can indicate hilar lymphadenopathy. The endoscope should be manipulated throughout all the lobar bronchi and branches until it can no longer be safely advanced [41].

Once all lobes have been evaluated, bronchoalveolar lavage (BAL) should be performed in several different areas, including the lung appearing to be the most diseased. The author prefers BAL over transtracheal washes or bronchial brushings because it allows collection of fluid from a specific site and is thought to

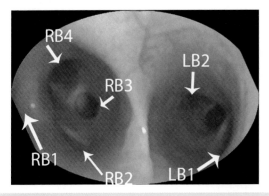

Fig. 4. Appearance of the carina during bronchoscopy. From this view, the branching pattern into lobar bronchi can be recognized. LB1, left cranial lobe; LB2, left caudal lung lobe; RB1, right cranial lung lobe; RB2, right middle lung lobe; RB3, accessory lung lobe; RB4, right caudal lung lobe.

represent the cells from the distal small airways and interstitium of the lung best. BAL is the only technique for which normal differential cell counts have been established for dogs and cats (Table 2) [41]. Because oral bacterial contamination can lead to false-positive culture results in BAL fluid, after gross visualization of the airways has been completed, the endoscope should be removed from the airways and cleaned by suctioning with sterile saline and air. The endoscope is then returned to the area chosen for BAL [41,42]. If no diseased area is recognized, the right middle lung lobe and caudal portion of the left cranial lung lobe are usually sampled because of their ventral orientation. BAL is performed when the scope is in a wedged position, and 10- to 20-mL aliquots of sterile saline are instilled into the airways depending on the size of the animal. The sample should then be immediately aspirated back into the same syringe, and a 40% to 90% return of the volume instilled can be expected. Lavage is generally performed twice in the same location, because greater fluid return is usually obtained on the second sample. The fluid can then be evaluated for total cell counts, cell differentials, cytology, and quantitative culture. Cytology not only helps to determine if inflammation is present but can aid in diagnosing infection, neoplasia, parasitic disease, or some fungal diseases. True bacterial infection is characterized by the presence of intracellular bacteria on cytology and bacterial growth of greater than 1.7×10^3 colony-forming units (CFUs) [43]. Smaller bacterial numbers are likely consistent with normal airway colonization.

DIAGNOSTICS FOR AIRWAY FUNCTION
Laryngoscopy
Laryngoscopy allows direct visualization of the larynx and associated structures and also provides the best assessment of laryngeal function. The cervical

Table 2
Differential cell counts from bronchoalveolar lavage fluid from normal dogs and cats

Study	Scott et al[a]	Rebar et al[b]	Padrid et al[c]	King et al[c]
Species	Canine	Canine	Feline	Feline
Number	46	9	24	11
Total cell count/mL	Not reported	516	303 ($\pm$126)	241 ($\pm$101)
% Macrophages	75 (27–92)	83	64 ($\pm$22)	70.6 ($\pm$9.8)
% PMNs	3 (0–30)	5	5 ($\pm$3)	6.7 ($\pm$4)
% Eosinophils	3 (3–28)	4.2	25 ($\pm$21)	16.1 ($\pm$6.8)
% Lymphs	10 (1–43)	5.7	4 ($\pm$3)	4.6 ($\pm$3.2)
% Mast cells	1 (0–5)	2.3	<1 ($\pm$<1)	Not reported
% Epithelial cells	Not reported	Not reported	2 ($\pm$ 2)	Not reported
% Goblet cells	Not reported	Not reported	<1 ($\pm$<1)	Not reported

Abbreviation: PMNs, polymorphonuclear cells.
[a]Values are median obtained from the second lavage performed in a lobe.
[b]Values are mean (range) from six lung lobes from all dogs.
[c]Values are mean ($\pm$SD) obtained from these cats.
Adapted from McKiernan BC. Bronchoscopy. In: McCarthy TC, editor. Veterinary endoscopy for the small animal practitioner. St. Louis: Elsevier; 2005. p. 224.

trachea can also be easily evaluated with a rigid 5-mm telescope to look for evidence of tracheal collapse. The normal laryngeal mucosa should be a light pink with readily visible blood vessels (Fig. 5). If laryngeal edema is present, the mucosa appears blanched and vessels are difficult to see. There should be minimal secretions within the larynx and cervical trachea in a normal dog or cat. The arytenoid cartilages should normally abduct symmetrically during inspiration. Dogs and cats with laryngeal paralysis show minimal to no abduction of the larynx on inspiration. It is imperative that the endoscopist be able to appreciate when the phase of inspiration occurs so as to confirm that abduction occurs at that time [41]. Laryngeal paralysis is most commonly bilateral in the dog and cat but can be unilateral [44]. It is well known that general anesthesia can dampen laryngeal movement, thus causing false-positive and false-negative diagnoses of laryngeal paralysis. It is suggested to use doxapram (Dopram-V) at a rate of 2.2 mg/kg administered intravenously during laryngoscopy to maximize laryngeal movement and to uncover any subtle changes in laryngeal function [45,46].

Arterial Blood Gas

An arterial blood gas measurement allows direct assessment of gas exchange, and thus is the most definitive assessment of overall pulmonary function. Most analyzers directly measure pH, PO_2, and PCO_2; HCO_3 and base excess are then calculated from these direct measurements. The femoral artery is most commonly used in dogs to obtain an arterial blood gas measurement, although alternatives include the dorsal metatarsal, carotid, brachial, and auricular

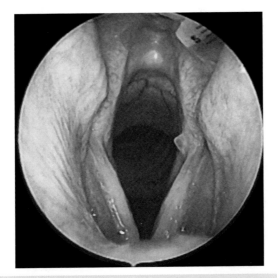

Fig. 5. Appearance of a normal canine larynx during laryngoscopy. The laryngeal mucosa should be light pink, with the blood vessels easily seen. The use of doxapram hydrogen chloride increases laryngeal movement to uncover subtle changes in laryngeal motion.

arteries [16,47]. Small-gauge needles (23–25 gauge) on 1- to 3-mL syringes are recommended, and a small volume of heparin (1000 U/mL) is drawn into the syringe to coat the needle hub and barrel. Arterial blood gas measurement in the cat is extremely difficult unless an indwelling catheter has been placed. To obtain an arterial sample in the canine patient, the patient should be placed in lateral recumbency. When using the femoral artery, the artery pulse is palpated with two fingers as high up in the inguinal area as possible. The needle is then directed into the palpated artery at an angle of 60°. Once a flash is seen within the hub of the needle, the needle should be kept completely still while the syringe is allowed to fill (if a preset syringe) or is aspirated back. It is best to use commercially available preset syringes that fill without aspiration and contain a filter through which air is displaced. These syringes also contain an anticoagulant to allow for the blood to be properly stored temporarily. To minimize any source of error, the sample should be kept on ice until analysis and analyzed as soon as possible [16,47,48].

The PO_2 obtained from an arterial blood sample (PaO_2) represents O_2 that is bound to hemoglobin and dissolved in the blood. PaO_2 in a normal animal at sea level should be greater than 80 mm Hg, although values are slightly lower at high altitudes. A decrease in PaO_2 can occur with hypoventilation, with a decrease in the partial pressure of atmospheric O_2 (high altitude), or with venous admixture. Venous admixture is perhaps the most common reason for hypoxemia and can occur with venous shunting (ie, lung atelectasis, pneumonia) or physiologic dead space (ie, PTE). If there is thickening of the lung interstitium, there can also be a diffusion barrier for O_2; however, this is fairly rare, given O_2's great reserve for diffusion [16,47,48].

As stated previously, hypoxemia can occur from high altitude or hypoventilation, neither of which is a cause of lung dysfunction. It is imperative when evaluating hypoxemia to compare the PaO_2 with the $PaCO_2$. The alveolar-arterial O_2 gradient gives an estimate of the effectiveness of gas transfer and is independent of the effect of ventilation. The gradient is calculated by first estimating the partial pressure of O_2 in the alveoli (PAO_2), using the alveolar gas equation:

$$PAO_2 = FIO_2(P_b - P_{H2O}) - PCO_2/RQ$$

where FIO_2 is the fractional inspired O_2 concentration, P_b is barometric pressure, P_{H2O} is the saturated water vapor pressure at body temperature, and RQ is the respiratory quotient (typically 0.9 at sea level). Measured arterial PaO_2 is then subtracted from the estimated alveolar PAO_2. Normal values in dogs are less than 10 to 15 mm Hg [13,16]. This equation includes the measurement of $PaCO_2$, and thus removes the possibility of hypoxemia induced by hypoventilation.

Pulmonary Lung Function Testing and Lung Mechanics

The function of the airways can be assessed by measuring resistance and compliance within the airways. Compliance (Cdyn) is the inverse of elastance, which is defined as the amount of elastic recoil within the lung. Cdyn is calculated as the change in lung volume divided by the change in transpulmonary pressure at two points of zero air flow. Resistance is a measurement that describes impedance to air flow, which is mostly frictional resistance of air currents against the walls of the airways. Resistance is defined as the pressure difference between the alveoli and the mouth divided by the flow rate of air [49].

Tidal breathing flow-volume loops (TBFVLs) were introduced into veterinary medicine to help bypass the need for patient cooperation or general anesthesia to evaluate air flow. Loops are generated by placing a pneumotachograph with a tight-fitting face mask over the patient's muzzle and measuring flow over time. The loops can then be evaluated for shape, respiratory rate, and tidal volume. Specific flow measurements and specific changes in the appearance of the loops can be obtained to help identify evidence of disease (Fig. 6). TBFVLs have been used in the diagnosis of laryngeal paralysis, brachycephalic syndrome, and chronic bronchitis in the dog [16,47,49]. For additional information on pulmonary function testing in small animal medicine, see the article by Hoffman elsewhere in this issue.

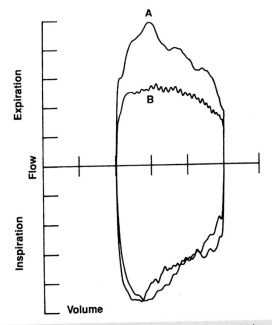

Fig. 6. A comparison of tidal breathing flow-volume loops (TBFVLs) obtained from a single healthy cat (A) and one bronchitic cat (B). Differences in expiratory flow (but not inspiratory flow) are readily apparent between the two loops. (*From* McKiernan BC, Dye JA, Rozanski EA. Tidal breathing flow-volume loops in healthy and bronchitic cats. J Vet Intern Med 1993:7(6):392; with permission.)

SUMMARY

The respiratory system provides many challenges by inherently being difficult to examine. The clinician must integrate history and physical examination findings to determine which diagnostic procedures are likely to be most effective in each case. Certain diagnostic tests (radiographs, CT, and bronchoscopy) provide extremely useful information when evaluating respiratory disease but do not provide any quantitative measurement of the disease. Other diagnostics (laryngoscopy, arterial blood gas, and TBFVLs) can help to quantify the degree of respiratory disease present.

References

[1] Nelson WA. Lower respiratory system. In: Slatter D, editor. Textbook of small animal surgery. 2nd edition. Philadelphia: WB Saunders; 1993. p. 800–3.

[2] Rivakumar P, Yilmaz C, Dane DM, et al. Regional lung growth following pneumonectomy assessed by computed tomography. J Appl Physiol 2004;97(4):1567–74.

[3] Corcoran B. Clinical evaluation of the patient with respiratory disease. In: Ettinger SJ, Feldman EC, editors. Textbook of veterinary internal medicine. 5th edition. Philadelphia: WB Saunders; 2000. p. 1034–9.

[4] Court MH, Dodman NH, Seeler DC. Inhalation therapy, oxygen administration, humidification, and aerosol therapy. VCNA 1985;15:1041–59.

[5] Schmidt-Nielson K, Bretz WL, Taylor CR. Panting in dogs: unidirectional air flow over evaporative surfaces. Science 1970;169:1102–4.

[6] Blatt CM, Taylor CR, Habel M. Thermal panting in dogs: the lateral nasal gland a source of water for evaporate cooling. Science 1972;177:804–5.

[7] Harpster NK. Physical examination of the respiratory tract. In: King LG, editor. Respiratory disease in dogs and cats. Philadelphia: WB Saunders; 2004. p. 67–72.

[8] Hedlund CS. Surgery of the upper respiratory system. In: Fossum TW, editor. Small animal surgery. St. Louis (MO): Mosby; 1997. p. 609–20.

[9] Schwartz AR, Smith PL, Kashima KH, et al. Respiratory function of the upper airways. In: Murray JF, Nadel JA, editors. 2nd edition. Textbook of respiratory medicine, vol. 2. Philadelphia: WB Saunders; 1994. p. 1451–70.

[10] Robinson NE. Airway physiology. VCNA 1992;22(5):1043–64.

[11] Guyton AC, Hall JE. Physical principles of gas exchange; diffusion of oxygen and carbon dioxide through the respiratory membrane. In: Guyton AC, editor. Textbook of medical physiology. 9th edition. Philadelphia: WB Saunders; 1996. p. 501–9.

[12] Rozanski E, Chan DL. Approach to the patient with respiratory distress. VCNA 2005;35: 307–17.

[13] West JB. Diffusion—how gas gets across the alveolar wall. In: Satterfield TS, editor. Respiratory physiology. 4th edition. Baltimore: Williams and Wilkins; 1990. p. 1–30.

[14] Rose BD, Post TW. Acid-base physiology. In: Clinical physiology of acid-base and electrolyte disorders. New York: McGraw-Hill; 2001. p. 299–325.

[15] Fuentes VL. Differential diagnosis of dyspnoea. In: Fuentes VL, Swift S, editors. BSAVA manual of small animal cardiorespiratory medicine and surgery. Cheltenham: BSAVA; 1998. p. 123–8.

[16] King LG, Hendricks JC. Clinical pulmonary function tests. In: Ettinger SJ, Feldman EC, editors. 4th edition. Textbook of veterinary internal medicine, vol. 1. Philadelphia: WB Saunders; 1995. p. 738–54.

[17] Hendricks JC. Brachycephalic airway syndrome. VCNA 1992;22(5):1145–54.

[18] Poncet CM, Dupre GP, Freiche VG, et al. Prevalence of gastrointestinal tract lesions in 73 brachycephalic dogs with upper respiratory syndrome. JSAP 2005;46(6):273–9.

[19] Gompf RE. Physical examination of the cardiopulmonary system. VCNA 1983;13(2):201–15.

[20] Lee JA, Drobatz KJ. Respiratory distress and cyanosis in dogs. In: King LG, editor. Respiratory disease in dogs and cats. Philadelphia: WB Saunders; 2004. p. 1–12.

[21] Maretta SM. Chronic rhinitis and dental disease. VCNA 1992;22(5):1101–18.

[22] Wolf AM. Fungal disease of the nasal cavity of the dog and cat. VCNA 1992;22(5): 1119–32.

[23] Forgacs P. Terminology. In: Lung sounds. London: Baillere Tindall; 1978. p. 1–6.

[24] Yeon S, Lee H, Change H, et al. Sound signature for identification of tracheal collapse and laryngeal paralysis in dogs. J Vet Med Sci 2005;67(1):91–5.

[25] Sigrist NE, Doherr MG, Spreng DE. Clinical findings and diagnostic value of posttraumatic thoracic radiographs in dogs and cats with blunt trauma. J Vet Emerg Crit Care 2000;14(4): 259–68.

[26] Center SA, Randolph JF, Erb HN, et al. Eosinophilia in the cat: a retrospective study of 312 cases (1975 to 1986). J Am Anim Hosp Assoc 1990;26(4):349–58.

[27] Bailiff NL, Norris CR. Clinical signs, clinicopathological findings, etiology, and outcome associated with hemoptysis in dogs: 36 cases (1990–1999). J Am Anim Hosp Assoc 2002;38(2):125–33.

[28] Legendre AM, Jacobs GJ, Green RT. Fungal disease (section III); blastomycoses, Cryptococcus, and coccidioidomycoses. In: Green RT, editor. Infectious diseases of the dog and cat. 2nd edition. Philadelphia: WB Saunders; 1998. p. 371–7, 383–90, 391–98.

[29] Saunders HM, Keith D. Thoracic imaging. In: King LG, editor. Respiratory disease in dogs and cats. Philadelphia: WB Saunders; 2004. p. 72–92.

[30] Thrall DE, Widmer WR. Radiation physics, radiation protection, and darkroom theory. In: Thrall DE, editor. Textbook of diagnostic veterinary radiology. 3rd edition. Philadelphia: WB Saunders; 1998. p. 1–19.

[31] Kneller SK. The larynx, pharynx, and trachea. In: Thrall DE, editor. Textbook of diagnostic veterinary radiology. 3rd edition. Philadelphia: WB Saunders; 1998. p. 263–8.

[32] Lamb CR. The canine lung. In: Thrall DE, editor. Textbook of diagnostic veterinary radiology. 3rd edition. Philadelphia: WB Saunders; 1998. p. 366–84.

[33] Reichle JK, Wisner ER. Non-cardiac thoracic ultrasound in 75 feline and canine patients. Vet Radiol Ultrasound 2000;41(2):154–62.

[34] Prather AB, Berry CR, Thrall DE. Use of radiography in combination with computed tomography for the assessment of noncardiac thoracic disease in the dog and cat. Vet Radiol Ultrasound 2005;46(2):114–21.

[35] Woodard PK, Sostman HD, MacFall JR, et al. Detection of pulmonary embolism: comparison of contrast-enhanced spiral CT and time-of-flight MR techniques. J Thorac Imaging 1995;10(1):59–72.

[36] Au JJ, Weisman DL, Stefanacci JD, et al. Use of computed tomography for evaluation of lung lesions associated with spontaneous pneumothorax in dogs: 12 cases. J Am Vet Med Assoc 2006;228(5):733–7.

[37] McCarthy TC. Rhinoscopy: the diagnostic approach to chronic nasal disease. In: McCarthy TC, editor. Veterinary endoscopy for the small animal practitioner. St. Louis (MO): Elsevier; 2005. p. 137–200.

[38] Norris AM, Laing EJ. Disease of the nose and sinuses. VCNA 1985;15(5):865–90.

[39] McCarthy TC, McDermaid SL. Rhinoscopy. VCNA 1990;20(5):1265–90.

[40] Amis T, McKiernan BC. Systematic identification of endobronchial anatomy during bronchoscopy in the dog. Am J Vet Res 1986;47:2649–57.

[41] McKiernan BC. Bronchoscopy. In: McCarthy TC, editor. Veterinary endoscopy for the small animal practitioner. St. Louis (MO): Elsevier; 2005. p. 201–38.

[42] Hawkins EC. Bronchoalveolar lavage. In: King LG, editor. Respiratory disease in dogs and cats. Philadelphia: WB Saunders; 2004. p. 118–27.

[43] Peeters DE, McKiernan BC, Weisiger RM, et al. Quantitative bacterial cultures and cytological examination of bronchoalveolar lavage specimens in dogs. J Vet Intern Med 2000;14: 534–41.

[44] Broome C, Burbridge HM, Pfeiffer DU. Prevalence of laryngeal paresis in dogs undergoing general anesthesia. Aust Vet J 2000;78:769–72.

[45] Miller CJ, McKiernan BC, Pace J, et al. The effects of doxapram hydrochloride (Dopram-V) on laryngeal function in healthy dogs. JVIM 2002;16(5):524–8.

[46] Tobias KM, Jackson AM, Harvey RC. Effects of doxapram HCl on laryngeal function of normal dogs and dogs with naturally occurring laryngeal paralysis. Vet Anaesth Analg 2004;31(4):258–63.

[47] McKiernan BC, Johnson LR. Clinical pulmonary function testing in dogs and cats. VCNA 1992;22(5):1087–100.

[48] Haskins SC. Interpretation of blood gas measurements. In: King LG, editor. Respiratory disease in dogs and cats. Philadelphia: WB Saunders; 2004. p. 181–92.

[49] Dye JA, Costa DL. Pulmonary mechanics. In: King LG, editor. Respiratory disease in dogs and cats. Philadelphia: WB Saunders; 2004. p. 157–74.

Advances in Respiratory Imaging

Eric G. Johnson, DVM*, Erik R. Wisner, DVM

Department of Surgical and Radiological Sciences, School of Veterinary Medicine,
Veterinary Medical Teaching Hospital Small Animal Clinic, University of California at Davis,
1 Shields Avenue, Davis, CA 95616, USA

Imaging for the diagnosis of respiratory disease has routinely involved conventional radiography of the affected area. With the expanded availability of CT, this modality has demonstrated its usefulness in enhancing the sensitivity and specificity of respiratory imaging as a diagnostic tool. This article focuses on some of the newer approaches to imaging diagnoses and introduces the tomographic features of common respiratory disorders.

SINONASAL DISORDERS

Equipment and Technique

Radiographic studies of the nasal cavity and associated paranasal sinuses should include lateral and open- and closed-mouth ventrodorsal views to assess the nasal cavity fully, oblique projections to evaluate the osseous boundaries of the nasal cavity and paranasal sinuses, and a rostrocaudal projection to highlight the frontal sinuses. Animals must be under general anesthesia to achieve these views. At the authors' institution, all radiographic studies are acquired using a digital radiographic system (Eklin digital radiographic plate with Cannon image processing software, Eklin Medical Systems, Inc., Santa Clara, California) and resulting images are viewed on 3-megapixel gray-scale monitors. High-detail film screen combinations are also an excellent method for obtaining diagnostic nasal radiographs.

With the relatively recent advances in CT technology and design, the time required to complete studies has decreased dramatically. In fact, the time required to complete a CT scan of the nasal cavity is usually less than that required to perform conventional skull radiographs. At the authors' institution, a single-slice helical CT scanner (GE HiSpeed Advantage x/i; GE Medical Systems, Milwaukee, Wisconsin) is used. Patients are anesthetized and positioned in sternal recumbency, and 3- to 7-mm helical images (120 kV, 100 mA) of the skull are acquired from the tip of the nasal planum to the retropharyngeal lymph nodes. Images are viewed in stack mode on a workstation and evaluated

*Corresponding author. E-mail address: egjohnson@ucdavis.edu (E.G. Johnson).

0195-5616/07/$ – see front matter
doi:10.1016/j.cvsm.2007.05.004

in a wide bone window (window width = 2500, window level = 480) as well as in a narrow soft tissue window (window width = 340, widow level = 25). Thinner images (1–2-mm collimation) are often acquired to evaluate abnormalities detected on the initial images more fully. Intravenous contrast material can be useful in determining the extent and pattern of contrast enhancement of a nasal lesion. For neoplastic nasal masses, contrast media administration is also used to help further delineate tumor margins and to assess lymph nodes for evidence of regional metastasis.

Inflammatory Nasal Disorders

Foreign body rhinitis

Radiographic diagnosis of nasal foreign bodies depends on whether the object is radiopaque. Wood or grass foreign bodies are not directly identified, and radiographic findings are often minimal [1]. Radiopaque foreign bodies are not usually a diagnostic challenge; however, orthogonal radiographic projections are needed to confirm anatomic location accurately. Chronic nasal foreign bodies may result in radiographic evidence of unilateral increased soft tissue opacity or in focal destructive rhinitis [1].

CT seems to be more sensitive and specific than radiographic studies for diagnosis of nasal foreign bodies. CT characteristics of nasal foreign bodies may include direct visualization of the foreign body, evidence of localized turbinate destruction, or minimal to moderate localized soft tissue opacity surrounding the foreign body [2]. CT also provides a detailed map of the nasal passages to guide rhinoscopic nasal foreign body retrieval.

Fungal rhinitis

The typical radiographic features of canine nasal aspergillosis have been defined as loss of turbinate architecture, especially rostrally, and thickening of the frontal bone [3]. Frontal sinus involvement is variable and is often identified as soft tissue density within the frontal sinuses.

The CT features of canine nasal aspergillosis have been described as destruction of the nasal turbinates with resulting cavitation of the affected nasal passage; focal or regional accumulation of abnormal soft tissue in the nasal passages; thickening of the mucosa of the frontal sinus, nasal cavity, and maxillary recess; and thickened reactive bone [4]. In many dogs, fungal granulomas of mixed gas and soft tissue opacity are present in the frontal sinus or caudal nasal cavity. In a few affected dogs, erosive bone destruction may also be evident, which can mimic the appearance of nasal neoplasia. Early in the course of disease, imaging findings are almost always unilateral with extension to the ipsilateral frontal sinus. Later in the disease process, the contralateral nasal cavity and frontal sinus may also be affected, although the disease remains unilateral in most dogs [4]. This constellation of CT features is highly characteristic of aspergillosis, and a diagnosis is highly suspected based on CT imaging findings alone. It has been shown that CT is far more sensitive than radiography for the detection and diagnosis of canine nasal aspergillosis lesions (Fig. 1) [5].

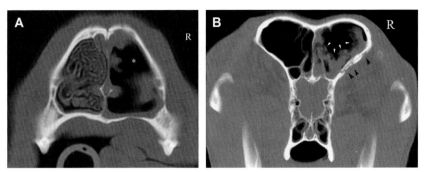

Fig. 1. (A) CT image at the level of the third maxillary premolar in a 4-year-old mixed-breed dog with a history of unilateral mucoid nasal discharge demonstrates cavitary destruction of the right nasal turbinates (*) with a region of abnormal soft tissue opacification affecting the right nasal passage. (B) CT image at the level of the frontal sinuses reveals thickened mucosa with mixed amorphous gas and soft tissue opacity within the right frontal sinus (*white arrows*). Additionally, there is a mixed productive and destructive bony change associated with the ventral floor of the right frontal sinus (*black arrowheads*). These findings are highly suggestive of nasal aspergillosis, which was confirmed with rhinoscopy and histopathologic examination.

Feline fungal rhinitis is most often attributable to infection with *Cryptococcus* rather than *Aspergillus* species. *Cryptococcus neoformans* is saprophytic yeast and is the most common systemic mycotic infectious organism in cats. Typically, this organism produces a hyperplastic rather than destructive rhinitis [6]. If fungal granulomas form in later stages of the disease, however, these may expand to destroy nasal turbinates and paranasal bones. *Aspergillus* rhinitis is rare in cats and may appear as a destructive rhinitis with radiographic and CT features similar to those of canine aspergillosis. Imaging features include profound destruction of the turbinate bones, increased soft tissue density in the nasal cavity, and frontal and sphenoid sinus fluid accumulation [7].

Nonspecific rhinitis in the dog
Nonspecific rhinitis is a general term encompassing inflammatory nasal conditions. Radiographs can be normal or range from a unilateral or bilateral increase in opacity within the nasal passages. The paranasal sinuses may or may not be involved [1].

The CT changes of nonspecific rhinitis are typically mild, although cases vary in severity and laterality. They may include a bilateral nondestructive process with minimal to marked mucosal thickening and nasal fluid accumulation. Occasionally, there may be minimal to moderate fluid accumulation in the frontal sinuses and mild or moderate turbinate destruction, typically without overt destruction of cortical bone forming nasal cavity and sinus boundaries [2].

Canine nasal neoplasia
Many types of tumors can arise within the canine nasal cavity, largely because of the many different cell types in this area. The most common nasal tumors are carcinomas, with adenocarcinoma being the most common. Definitive

diagnosis of nasal neoplasia requires biopsy, but imaging features of nasal neoplasia may lead to a presumptive diagnosis with a high degree of confidence. Radiographic signs of nasal neoplasia include erosion of the facial bones and vomer bones in addition to destruction of the normal turbinate pattern with increased soft tissue opacity within the nasal passages [1,8]. Frontal sinus involvement, appearing as fluid opacity replacing the normal air-filled cavities, is often identified secondary to obstruction of the nasofrontal aperture or secondary to direct extension of the tumor into one or both frontal sinuses.

CT is far more sensitive than conventional radiography for the detection of abnormalities of the nasal passages and skull attributable to nasal neoplasia in dogs [9]. CT allows for a more complete evaluation of the nasal cavity, endoturbinates and ectoturbinates, retrobulbar space, cribriform plate, frontal sinuses, and associated structures by removing superimposition of adjacent structures. Common CT findings of nasal neoplasia include ethmoid bone destruction, destruction of the nasal bone or maxilla, abnormal soft tissue in the retrobulbar space, moderate to severe turbinate destruction, frontal sinus fluid with soft tissue accumulation, a mass-like lesion in the nasal cavity, and patchy areas of increased attenuation within a soft tissue density (Fig. 2) [2,10]. CT also provides excellent guidance for rhinoscopy and nasal biopsy collection. Occasionally, if a large enough defect is identified in the nasal or paranasal bones using CT, ultrasound guidance can be used to obtain core biopsies of intranasal or perinasal masses.

Contrast medium uptake may be extremely nonuniform and frequently does not delineate tumor margins accurately. Because the CT features described often lead to a presumptive diagnosis of nasal neoplasia, the authors administer

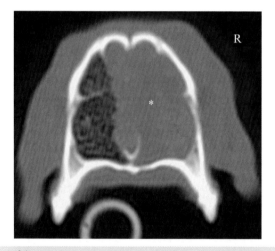

Fig. 2. CT image of the nasal cavity in a 10-year-old Sheltie presented with a 2-month history of right nasal epistaxis reveals a mass lesion in the right nasal cavity with destruction of the nasal septum and underlying nasal turbinates (*). Histopathologic examination confirmed nasal carcinoma.

intravenous iodinated contrast media to delineate tumor margins only when a breach of the paranasal bones has occurred. This helps to determine whether frontal sinus opacity is attributable to extension of nasal tumor or secondary to obstructive rhinitis. In the authors' experience, if complete opacification of one or both frontal sinuses is present, there is a high likelihood of nasal neoplasia. If the cribriform plate is disrupted, the degree of neoplastic extension into the calvarium can be more accurately assessed after administration of contrast. Contrast material administration can also help to evaluate the enhancement pattern of regional lymph nodes.

It is not possible to differentiate carcinoma from sarcoma based on radiographic or CT findings because they share many imaging characteristics. Definitive diagnosis of nasal neoplasia requires biopsy with histopathologic examination. Sarcomas of the nasal passages include chondrosarcomas, osteosarcomas, and multilobular osteochondrosarcomas as well as soft tissue sarcomas. Tumors that arise from the paranasal bones are more likely to be osteosarcomas or multilobular osteochondrosarcomas (Fig. 3). Chondrosarcomas typically appear aggressive and invasive, with regions of paranasal bone lysis. Spicules of mineralization can often be identified dissecting through these mass lesions.

Canine nasal lymphoma, although uncommon, has been documented multiple times at the authors' institution. Lymphoma can mimic the radiographic and CT findings of carcinomas and sarcomas, but its appearance is often less aggressive. CT features may include mild to moderate soft tissue opacification of the nasal passages, minimal turbinate destruction, and small multifocal nodules adjacent to turbinates. More aggressive appearing lesions are also possible,

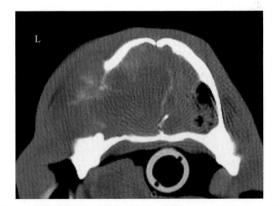

Fig. 3. CT image of a 7-year-old Pit Bull Terrier presented with unilateral epistaxis and swelling of the left side of the muzzle. This image illustrates a primarily destructive lesion centered around the left nasal and maxillary bone. There is a soft tissue mass effect in the left nasal cavity that extends through the nasal septum into the right nasal passage. Irregular new bone formation is identified around the left nasal bone within the associated soft tissue mass. Histopathologic examination was diagnostic for nasal osteosarcoma.

including large space-occupying nasal masses with associated bone loss. Nasopharyngeal soft tissue masses or polypoid lesions also are a common concurrent feature and may be the only significant CT finding. Adjacent lymph node enlargement is often not a concurrent feature (Fig. 4).

Feline sinonasal disease

Unlike the imaging findings in dogs, radiographic features of feline chronic rhinitis and sinonasal neoplasia are similar. Nasal carcinoma is a commonly reported neoplasm in the cat [11], although recent studies report lymphoma as a common tumor type as well [12,13]. Radiographic features reported with chronic rhinitis and nasal neoplasia include opacification of the frontal sinuses and nasal cavity; loss of definition of the nasal turbinates; a soft tissue mass effect; bony changes, including erosions of the paranasal bones, nasal septum, and nasal conchae; and deviation of the nasal septum. Radiographic changes more suggestive of feline nasal neoplasia than rhinitis include unilateral lysis of the paranasal bones, unilateral nasal turbinate destruction, and loss of teeth [13].

In feline nasal disease, CT is more sensitive than radiographs for detecting nasal cavity disorders and is more accurate for determining the anatomic extent of disease. CT abnormalities in nasal neoplasia are quite similar to the CT findings in chronic nasal disease, however, thus making nasal biopsy necessary for diagnosis. CT findings in both disease processes include deviation of the nasal septum, cribriform plate destruction, turbinate destruction, frontal sinus involvement, destruction of the paranasal bones, and involvement of extrasinonasal structures. Feline nasal neoplasia and inflammatory nasal diseases often

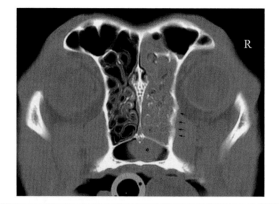

Fig. 4. CT image of a 3-year-old Rhodesian Ridgeback dog with a history of sneezing, stertor, and nasal discharge. There is soft tissue–attenuating material dissecting through the right ethmoturbinates and extending into the right frontal sinus. There is mild osteolysis of the vertical portion of the frontal bone (*black arrows*). A soft tissue polypoid mass can be seen within the nasopharyngeal meatus (*). Immunocytochemistry of fine needle aspirates was diagnostic for B-cell lymphoma.

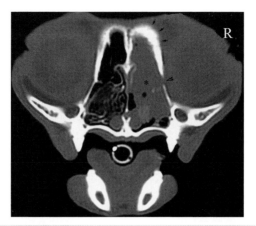

Fig. 5. CT image at the level of the orbits in an 8-year-old Scottish Fold presented with a history of chronic sneezing and nasal discharge shows soft tissue opacification of the right nasal passage with underlying turbinate loss (*). There is hyperostosis of the dorsal maxillary bone (*arrows*) with osteolysis of bone at the junction of the maxillary bone with the lacrimal bone (*arrowhead*). Rhinoscopy and biopsy demonstrated chronic neutrophilic and lymphoplasmacytic rhinitis.

involve both nasal cavities (Fig. 5) [12]. CT findings more suggestive of feline sinonasal neoplasia include bony change of the maxillary, lacrimal, and palatine bones; severe maxilloturbinate destruction; and pathologic changes of the facial soft tissues and orbit by extension. Also, identification of a homogeneous space-occupying mass with destruction of the nasal septum is highly suggestive of nasal neoplasia (Fig. 6) [12].

THORAX
Conventional film radiology continues to be the mainstay of thoracic imaging. With the advent of helical CT technology, however, CT has become an important adjunct to the diagnostic evaluation of thoracic disorders. In general, CT provides better lesion characterization and delineation than conventional radiography for many thoracic disorders. Recognizing that thoracic radiography is the first diagnostic imaging step for patients with thoracic disease, the remainder of this section focuses on CT imaging features of commonly encountered thoracic disorders.

THORACIC CT
Equipment
Thoracic CT is best performed on third- or fourth-generation helical machines using a forced single-breath-hold helical scanning technique. Multiple detector arrays are now available that greatly reduce scan times; however, single detector arrays are adequate and often more economically feasible. At the authors' institution, images are obtained on a single-slice helical CT scanner (GE

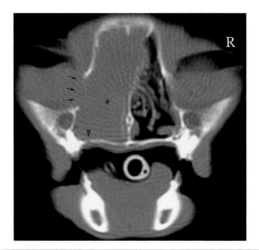

Fig. 6. CT image at the level of the rostral zygomatic arch in a 13-year-old domestic short-haired cat presented with a history of nasal discharge and sneezing demonstrates a homogeneous space-occupying mass with destruction of the nasal septum (*). Destruction is identified at the junction of the maxillary, lacrimal, and frontal bones (*arrows*). Subtle destruction is also identified involving the palatine bone (*arrowhead*). Rhinoscopy with histopathologic examination was diagnostic for nasal lymphoma.

HiSpeed Advantage x/i). Animals are placed under general anesthesia and are maintained in dorsal or ventral recumbency to avoid atelectasis, which often occurs if the patients are transported to the CT gantry in lateral recumbency. The patients are manually hyperventilated just before the helical scan to decrease inspiratory drive during the forced breath hold. Contiguous helical images of the entire thorax are acquired using a slice collimation of 3 to 7 mm depending on the size of the patient. The slice thickness is chosen to allow the thorax to be scanned under a single breath hold that does not exceed 50 to 60 seconds. Images are evaluated in stack mode on a workstation in a lung window (window width = 2000, window level = 650) and a mediastinal window (window width = 750, window level = 70). When necessary, thinner slices are obtained through regions of pathologic findings recognized on the initial scan.

Mediastinal and Pleural Space Disorders

Mediastinal masses

Mediastinal masses can be localized to the cranial, middle, or caudal reflection of the mediastinum. Common mediastinal masses include thymoma, lymphoma, mediastinal cysts, and, occasionally, sarcomas. Often, radiographs in conjunction with ultrasonographic interrogation of the region are diagnostic for the presence of a mass or cyst. Conventional radiography and ultrasound are poorly sensitive for determining if a mediastinal lesion is aggressive with respect to vascular invasion; displacement of normal mediastinal structures (eg, vasculature, esophagus); and invasion of adjacent structures, such as the thoracic wall or adjacent lung, however. For these reasons, CT is the method of choice for evaluating mediastinal masses in people [14]. In dogs and cats, CT of the mediastinum is useful for surgical planning, specifically for determining approximate tumor margins and the presence and extent of vascular invasion and to evaluate for nonradiographically apparent spread of disease, such as regional lymph node or pulmonary metastasis [15].

Chylothorax

Chylothorax is a condition characterized by accumulation of chyle within the pleural space that leads to respiratory impairment. Although chylothorax manifests as a pleural space disease, it results from pathologic change associated with the thoracic duct or its tributaries that reside within the mediastinum. In patients with chronic chylothorax, radiographs typically reveal variable amounts of pleural effusion, reduction in lung lobe volume, rounding of the lobar margins, and pleural thickening. In patients with idiopathic chylothorax, imaging of the thoracic duct is typically performed before surgical intervention. In veterinary medicine, this has traditionally been performed by surgical catheterization of an intestinal lymphatic vessel, followed by fluoroscopic and radiographic examination during lymphatic injection of iodinated contrast material. This technique is useful for defining the inherently variable anatomy of the thoracic duct and for demonstrating the location and character of the ductal lesion [16].

Recently, several studies have been performed to define the CT imaging characteristics of the canine thoracic duct. One study used traditional catheterization of a mesenteric lymphatic vessel and subsequent injection of iodinated contrast material to opacify the thoracic duct. This study was performed in normal dogs and suggested that CT can be used to define the number and location of thoracic duct branches more accurately than traditional radiographic lymphangiography [17]. Another study performed in dogs with presumed idiopathic chylothorax used a closed abdominal technique for opacification of the thoracic duct before thoracic CT. This technique involved direct lymphangiography by means of ultrasound-guided mesenteric lymph node injection of nonionic iodinated contrast material to achieve thoracic duct opacification. This technique provides excellent contrast enhancement of the thoracic duct and has documented dilated, tortuous, cranial mediastinal lymphatics that seem to be similar to idiopathic cranial mediastinal lymphangiectasia (Fig. 7) [18].

Pyothorax

Pyothorax is typically diagnosed in an animal with radiographic evidence of pleural effusion by performing pleural fluid analysis and culture. Radiographic features include unilateral or bilateral pleural fluid accumulation, reduction of aerated lung volume, and rounding or thickening of pleural margins. Occasionally, pleural adhesions involving the thoracic wall or diaphragm may occur [1]. Real or apparent alveolar pulmonary infiltrates may occur in patients with concurrent foreign body migration, pulmonary abscessation, or atelectasis. Pleural

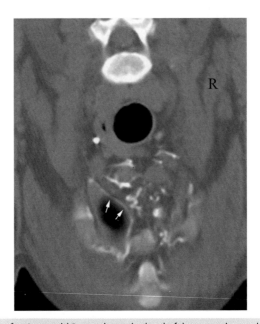

Fig. 7. CT image of a 4-year-old Rottweiler at the level of the second sternebral segment after mesenteric lymph node injection with iodinated contrast material. There is excellent opacification of dilated cranial mediastinal lymphatic vessels consistent with idiopathic cranial mediastinal lymphangiectasia. Contrast material is present in the pleural space surrounding the left cranial lung lobe consistent with leakage from a mediastinal lymph vessel or vessels (*arrows*).

fluid often obscures thoracic structures, and repeat radiographic examination after removal of the fluid can be useful in evaluating the pulmonary parenchyma and cardiac silhouette.

CT may be indicated in patients with pyothorax that do not respond to conventional management techniques and in patients in which a pleural or pulmonary foreign body or abscess is suspected. Because of the cross-sectional nature of CT, superimposition and silhouetting of structures caused by loculated or residual pleural fluid are eliminated. CT findings associated with pyothorax include pleural and mediastinal fluid accumulation, encapsulated fluid accumulation (pleural abscess), thickening and rounding of pleural margins, thickening of mediastinal pleura, mild to moderate mediastinal and hilar lymphadenopathy (more significant with fungal organisms), pulmonary atelectasis, pulmonary alveolar infiltrates, and, occasionally, pleural adhesions.

CT can also reveal a pulmonary abscess, which typically appears as a thick-walled fluid-filled structure that may contain a gas-fluid interface. It can be difficult to differentiate an infected neoplasm from a primary pulmonary abscess. Chronic foreign bodies may lead to pulmonary abscessation, (Fig. 8) or may appear as focal regions of alveolar infiltrates surrounded by bronchiectatic airways.

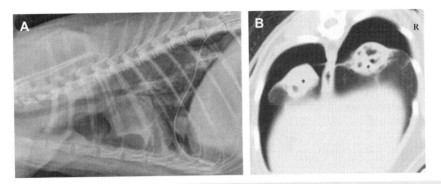

Fig. 8. Images from a 2-year-old cat with a history of pyothorax that was nonresponsive to chest tube placement and antibiotic therapy. (A) Right lateral thoracic radiograph reveals thickening of the pleural surface with small regions of plural fluid accumulation and a small volume of free pleural gas. There is a chest tube placed in the caudal thorax. A region of alveolar opacity is identified within the caudal mediastinum just behind the cardiac silhouette. Within the caudodorsal lung fields is a well-circumscribed alveolar opacity with overlying gas opacity suggestive of a pulmonary abscess. This alveolar density was difficult to identify on the orthogonal projections. (B) CT image of the caudal thorax of the same cat. Two well-circumscribed alveolar densities with central gas opacities are identified at the periphery of the left and right caudal lung lobes (*). There is thickening of the adjacent pleural surfaces and pneumothorax. Surgery revealed compartmentalized caudal mediastinal and pleural fluid with pleuritis and focal abscessation of the right and left caudal lung lobes. Histopathologic examination revealed chronic, necrotizing and suppurative bronchopneumonia with foreign material and fibrosis and chronic necrosuppurative pleuritis with granulation tissue.

In patients with pyothorax undergoing contrast CT, pleural surfaces are often moderately to markedly contrast enhancing because of the marked thickening, hyperemia, and increased vascular permeability of the pleura. Pleural abscesses often appear as ring-enhancing cystic masses with a fluid-attenuating core, although central attenuation may be significantly higher (30–60 Hounsfield units) because of the cellular and protein content of abscess fluid. Mediastinal and tracheobronchial lymph nodes may also be easier to identify and differentiate from surrounding tissues on contrast-enhanced CT studies. Nodes tend to be moderately to markedly contrast enhancing and should generally have a uniform pattern of contrast enhancement. A central contrast void may be recognized that corresponds to fat within the lymph node hilus.

Pneumothorax

Pneumothorax can result from trauma, foreign body migration, rupture of a pulmonary bulla or subpleural bleb, iatrogenic causes, visceral pleural erosion from underlying inflammatory lung disease, or necrosing neoplasia. Although pneumothorax is readily diagnosed using conventional radiography, the inciting abnormality is not easily recognized in patients, with the exception of traumatic and iatrogenic pneumothorax. Because the underlying cause of pneumothorax has an impact on treatment and prognosis, CT is often indicated in this subset of patients.

Spontaneous pneumothorax can be caused by rupture of a pulmonary bulla or subpleural bleb [19]. A bulla is defined as a region of vesicular emphysema located within the pulmonary parenchyma. A bleb is a thin-walled gas-filled structure that is located subpleurally and often arises as a sequela of air dissection from damaged alveoli [1,20]. Radiographically, bullae are characterized by a region of hyperlucency within the pulmonary parenchyma that may or may not include a thin rim of surrounding tissue. Blebs are similar in appearance to bullae; however, they are typically located at the apices of the lung and are subpleural [1]. Radiographic detection of blebs and bullae in dogs ranges from 0% to 50% [20]. This is likely attributable to superimposition of overlying anatomy surrounding a small gas-filled structure.

The CT findings associated with bullae and blebs in the dog include regions of low pulmonary parenchymal attenuation, disruption of the vascular pattern by pruning, and vascular distortion around areas of decreased attenuation (Fig. 9) [21]. Ruptured bullae and blebs often result in massive pneumothorax that may be unilateral or bilateral. Marked lung lobe atelectasis decreases lung volume, significantly increases pulmonary density, and obscures the underlying lesion. Patients undergoing CT for pneumothorax should have a chest tube placed before anesthesia to reduce the volume of pneumothorax and to reinflate an atelectatic lung. The pleural space should be evacuated and the study performed under mild positive-pressure ventilation to minimize atelectasis when possible. Although CT has been reported to be highly beneficial for the diagnosis of ruptured pulmonary bullae in patients with pneumothorax [21], in the authors' experience, CT has not been particularly rewarding in

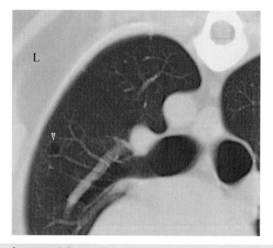

Fig. 9. CT image from an adult mixed-breed dog presented for a pulmonary mass. An incidental finding was a pulmonary bulla in the caudal subsegment of the left cranial lung lobe. Note the region of disrupted vasculature with a central region of hypoattenuation typical of pulmonary bullae (*arrowhead*).

localizing a ruptured bulla caused by persistent lobar atelectasis despite attempts to reinflate the lungs.

Airway-Oriented Disorders

Bronchial foreign bodies

Radiographic findings with bronchial foreign bodies are variable. If the foreign body is radiopaque, the diagnosis is often uncomplicated; however, diagnosis of radiolucent foreign bodies (eg, grass awns, sticks, wood) is not as simple. In the early stages of disease, radiographs of patients with nonradiopaque foreign bodies can appear normal. Radiographs become abnormal only after bronchial secretions accumulate or focal pneumonia develops. Common radiographic findings include focal interstitial pulmonary infiltrates with an accentuated bronchial pattern along a major bronchus, lobar or multifocal alveolar consolidations, focal bronchiectasis, pleural effusion with focal or multifocal pulmonary infiltrates, and pneumothorax (Fig. 10) [1].

The CT findings of bronchial foreign bodies are similar to the radiographic findings and include focal to multifocal (depending on the number of foreign bodies) interstitial to alveolar consolidations along an airway, focal lobar consolidation, focal bronchiectasis, pleural and mediastinal fluid accumulation, mild hilar and mediastinal lymphadenopathy, and pneumothorax. Given the superior contrast resolution of CT and its lack of superimposition of adjacent structures, nonradiopaque bronchial foreign bodies can occasionally be visualized.

Bronchial disease

Acute bronchial or tracheobronchial disease in the dog is usually radiographically subtle or silent. Architectural and cellular abnormalities must occur to result in clinically significant radiographic changes. These abnormalities include edema and cellular infiltration of the bronchial mucosa and submucosa, mucus covering the bronchial walls, proliferation and hyperplasia of bronchial linings, and inflammation of the peribronchial tissues [1]. The principal radiographic sign of canine chronic bronchitis has been described as bronchial wall thickening. This is seen radiographically as an increased number of thickened bronchi, visible end-on as "donuts" and as parallel lines in the long axis. Depending on the severity and chronicity of disease, additional radiographic signs may include bronchiectasis and interstitial infiltrates with obscuring of the pulmonary vasculature [1]. These radiographic signs are a sequela of bronchial mucosal edema, hyperplasia, mucus accumulation, and inflammation of the peribronchial tissues [22]. As normal dogs age, histopathologic changes are evident radiographically as a diffuse interstitial pattern, pleural thickening, and bronchial wall mineralization [23]. Some texts consider these radiographic findings similar to those in dogs with chronic bronchitis, and because many dogs with chronic bronchitis are older, some authors consider radiographs to be a nonspecific test for chronic bronchitis [1]. A recent study [24] found that the sensitivity of radiographs for the diagnosis of canine chronic bronchitis ranged from 52% to 65%, the specificity was 91%, and the accuracy ranged

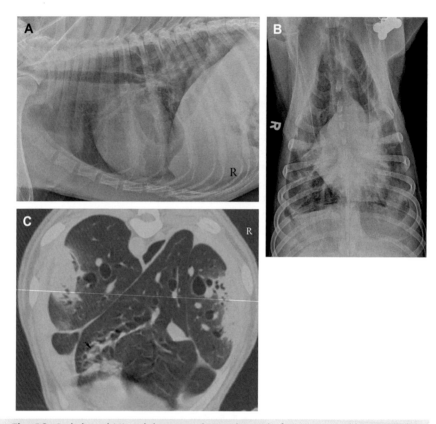

Fig. 10. Right lateral (A) and dorsoventral (B) radiographs from a 3-year-old German Short-Haired Pointer with a history of chronic cough. Interstitial to alveolar pulmonary infiltrates are identified within the left and right caudal lung lobes, right middle lung lobe, accessory lung lobe, and caudal subsegment of the left cranial lung lobe. Additionally, there are multiple focal regions of compartmentalized pleural effusion and thickening of the pleural surfaces. (C) Helical CT examination reveals multifocal regions of alveolar infiltrates within the right and left caudal lung lobes as well as in the accessory lung lobe. Multiple focal regions of bronchiectasis are also identified. A foreign body can be seen in the distal aspect of the accessory lung lobe (*arrow*). Bronchoscopy revealed multiple regions of bronchopneumonia with multiple grass awns within the airways and associated bronchiectasis.

from 65% to 74%. The most significant radiographic findings in that study supportive of chronic bronchitis were thickening of the bronchial walls and an increase in the number of bronchial wall shadows [24].

Thoracic CT may be much more accurate as an aid in the diagnosis of canine chronic bronchitis. By removing superimposing structures, individual bronchi can be more easily seen and more accurately characterized. Additionally, bronchial wall thickness can be directly measured on a computer workstation. Moreover, the peribronchial and interstitial tissues can be more accurately assessed for pathologic change.

Bronchiectasis is an airway-oriented condition characterized by persistent airway dilatation, often with suppuration. It is reported as a sequela to chronic uncontrolled infectious or inflammatory disease in dogs and cats. Radiographically, the disease can be recognized by thickened airway walls and dilated airways that fail to taper appropriately in the periphery. Focal pneumonia may also be present. In human and veterinary medicine, thoracic radiographs are insensitive for the diagnosis until late in the course of disease when irreversible changes have occurred. CT is the preferred method for diagnosis in human medicine, and the CT diagnosis of bronchiectasis is made using bronchial to adjacent pulmonary arterial diameter ratios. In the authors' experience in dogs with airway disease, a bronchial/arterial ratio of 2 or more is highly suggestive of bronchiectasis. Regions of increased interstitial pulmonary density can also be seen adjacent to the dilated bronchi (Fig. 11).

Feline airway disease
As with dogs, for pulmonary changes in cats to be evident radiographically, substantial cellular and architectural pulmonary changes must occur. In cats with chronic airway disease, these changes may include hyperplasia of the bronchial glands, bronchial wall cellular infiltration, hypertrophy of the bronchial smooth muscles, and, occasionally, bronchiectasis. Radiographic features of feline airway disease are similar to those in dogs and include increased

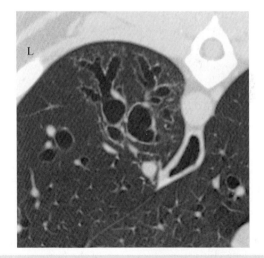

Fig. 11. CT image from an 8-year-old Labrador Retriever with a history of chronic cough and recurrent left caudal lung lobe infiltrates reveals focal bronchiectasis in the left caudal lung lobe with an irregular contour to the bronchial walls consistent with traction bronchiectasis. A ground-glass–like increase in interstitial pulmonary density is also identified adjacent to the dilated bronchi. Histopathologic examination of the affected lung revealed bronchiectasis, septal fibrosis, type II pneumocyte hyperplasia, alveolar histiocytosis, and lymphoplasmacytic peribronchitis. An underlying cause for the lesion was not determined, but it was most consistent with a previous pneumonia.

radiodensity and thickening of bronchial walls, increased visibility and numbers of bronchial markings, increased peribronchial radiodensity, a diffuse increase in interstitial pulmonary radiodensity, soft tissue accumulation in airways suggestive of mucus plugging, hyperinflation, collapse of the right middle lung lobe, and occasional bronchiectasis (Fig. 12) [1].

The CT findings in feline airway disease are similar to the radiographic features; however, given the lack of superimposition, this modality is likely more sensitive than conventional radiography. Soft tissue material deposited in airways (suggestive of mucus plugging) is more obvious with CT. Interstitial markings may appear multifocal and coalescing, and these opacities can resemble the ground-glass appearance that has been reported to represent active alveolitis or fibrosis in people (Fig. 13) [25]. Linear, parenchymal, soft tissue opacities that are nontapering and peripheral (similar to parenchymal bands identified in human beings) are also occasionally seen. These are thought to represent areas of atelectasis or fibrosis (Fig. 14) [26].

Pulmonary Parenchymal Disorders
Pulmonary masses
Conventional radiography is often used to identify thoracic masses but may be less useful for differentiating pulmonary, mediastinal, or thoracic wall origin and for localizing a pulmonary mass to a specific lung lobe. In addition, CT provides more accurate assessment of the likelihood of an inflammatory versus a neoplastic mass and for detecting mediastinal and hilar lymph node involvement [27]. Additional information provided by CT compared with traditional radiography includes defining mediastinal or pulmonary location of masses, the extent of lung pathologic change with delineation of lung versus pleural masses,

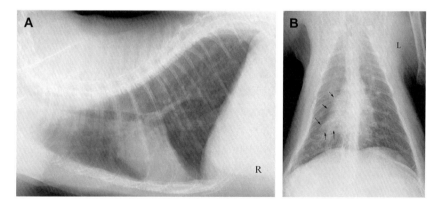

Fig. 12. Lateral (A) and dorsoventral (B) radiographs of a 3-year-old domestic short-haired cat with a history of coughing. There is a diffuse bronchial pattern with airway thickening identified in all lung fields. The patient is hyperinflated, and there is right middle lung lobe collapse (*arrows in B*). There is a diffuse increase in interstitial pulmonary radiodensity. The diagnosis was chronic airway disease.

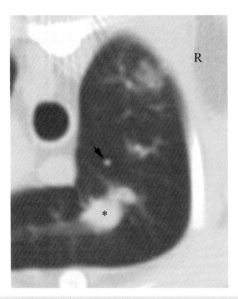

Fig. 13. CT image of a 5-year-old cat with a history of chronic coughing shows a large soft tissue density in the right cranial lung lobe bronchus consistent with an intraluminal mucus plug (*). A smaller mucus plug is seen immediately dorsally (*arrow*). Additionally, there are ground-glass pulmonary opacities present in the dorsal aspect of the right cranial lung suggestive of active alveolitis or fibrosis. These findings are consistent with chronic active airway disease.

the location of cavitated lung nodules, and the detection of bony lesions or pulmonary metastasis (Fig. 15) [15].

CT has been shown to be far more sensitive than conventional radiography for detecting pulmonary metastatic neoplasia in people [28]. Similarly, in dogs, only 9% of nodules detected with CT were identifiable on comparable thoracic radiographs [29]. CT allows detection of nodules that measure 1 mm in diameter versus conventional radiographs in which nodules must reach 7 to 9 mm before they are consistently detected (Fig. 16).

Alveolar pulmonary disease

An alveolar pulmonary pattern is caused by displacement of air from the pulmonary parenchyma. The radiographic characteristics of an alveolar pattern include air bronchogram formation; soft tissue opacification of lung; lobar consolidation; and silhouetting of adjacent soft tissue structures, including the heart and pulmonary vessels. The common disease processes associated with this pattern are bronchopneumonia, neoplasia, severe edema, and pulmonary hemorrhage.

CT can prove valuable in patients with chronic alveolar pulmonary consolidation that is nonresponsive to conventional therapies. It may reveal pulmonary masses obscured by overlying alveolar disease or small pulmonary nodules not visualized with conventional radiography [27,29]. Additionally,

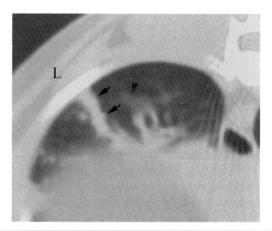

Fig. 14. CT image of the thorax of a young adult cat with a history of chronic coughing. There is a linear, nontapering, parenchymal soft tissue opacity in the left caudal lung lobe suggestive of fibrosis and scarring from associated chronic airway disease (*arrows*). Additionally, bronchial wall thickening and ground-glass opacities (*arrowhead*) are present, suggesting active alveolitis or fibrosis.

bronchial foreign bodies or pulmonary architectural abnormalities, such as bronchiectasis, that predispose patients to chronic recurrent pneumonia may be recognized. The peribronchial lymph nodes also can be more accurately assessed because they are better visualized with CT than with conventional radiography.

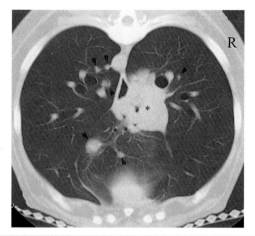

Fig. 15. CT image from an 11-year-old mixed-breed dog with a solitary pulmonary mass evident radiographically demonstrates a well-circumscribed pulmonary mass at the junction of the right caudal lung lobe bronchus and the accessory lung lobe bronchus (*). Additionally, several well-circumscribed pulmonary nodules are visible in multiple lung fields (*arrowheads*). Histopathologic examination revealed pulmonary adenocarcinoma with intrapulmonary metastases.

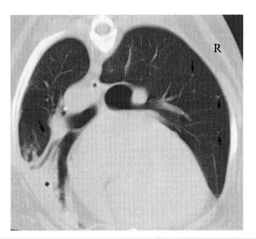

Fig. 16. Helical CT image of a 12-year-old Collie with a bleeding splenic mass demonstrates multiple soft tissue nodules within the pulmonary parenchyma (*arrows*). Atelectasis is noted in the caudal subsegment of the left cranial lung lobe (*), illustrating the need for a forced breath hold to avoid obscuring pulmonary pathologic findings. Histopathologic examination revealed splenic hemangiosarcoma with pulmonary metastases to the lungs.

Diffuse pulmonary disease

The CT characteristics of diffuse pulmonary disease are not well described in the veterinary literature. Caution should be exercised in drawing too many parallels with CT patterns described in human beings because of the anatomic differences in the subgross lung anatomy of dogs and cats.

Canine idiopathic pulmonary fibrosis

Interstitial lung disease is a poorly understood and characterized disease in the dog and cat [30]. Canine idiopathic pulmonary fibrosis (CIPF) is most apparent in middle-aged to geriatric dogs and seems to be overrepresented in West Highland White Terriers [31]. Alveolar septal thickening seems to be the predominant change identified histopathologically [30,31]. Radiographic findings include a diffuse interstitial pattern that sometimes may be miliary. Lung fields often appear to be hypoinflated secondary to decreased pulmonary compliance. Occasionally, right heart enlargement and associated pulmonary arterial enlargement can be identified as a sequela to secondary pulmonary hypertension (Fig. 17).

Recently high-resolution CT has been used to evaluate suspected cases of CIPF [32]. Unfortunately, only small numbers of dogs have CT images and concurrent histopathologic confirmation of CIPF. CT findings considered consistent with CIPF include ground-glass opacity, traction bronchiectasis, interstitial thickening, and honeycombing [32]. Ground-glass opacity is defined as an increase in lung opacity that does not obscure underlying vessels. This finding may indicate active alveolar inflammation or fibrosis [33]. Traction bronchiectasis is characterized by bronchial dilation with an irregular contour.

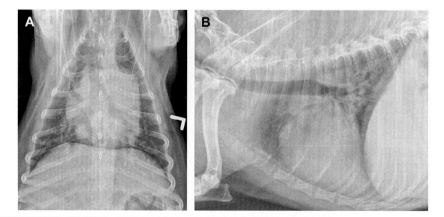

Fig. 17. Right lateral (A) and dorsoventral (B) radiographs of a 13-year-old terrier cross presented with a history of tachypnea. There is a diffuse heavy interstitial pattern with a mild underlying bronchial pattern. These radiographs were taken at maximum inspiration, and the patient is hypoinflated, suggesting decreased pulmonary compliance. There is moderate right heart enlargement with mildly enlarged pulmonary arteries. Necropsy with histopathologic examination revealed extensive multifocal primary interstitial pulmonary fibrosis with right heart hypertrophy suggesting secondary pulmonary hypertension.

It is thought to result from traction on the bronchial wall secondary to fibrosis of the lung parenchyma [34]. Honeycombing is defined by cystic air-filled spaces several millimeters in diameter that are often peripheral, and in human medicine, this indicates dissolution of alveoli and loss of architecture [32].

Coccidioidomycosis

Coccidioidomycosis is caused by *Coccidioides immitis,* a dimorphic fungus endemic to the southwestern United States. The most frequent primary site of infection is the lung. The radiographic features of coccidioidomycosis are similar to those of other fungal diseases and include peribronchial, micronodular pulmonary lesions (miliary pulmonary pattern), ill-defined pulmonary consolidations, or occasional lobar consolidations. Tracheobronchial and mediastinal lymphadenopathy is a common feature [1].

The CT features of pulmonary coccidioidomycosis are similar to the radiographic features. Tracheobronchial and mediastinal lymphadenopathy are easier to identify with CT because of the removal of superimposed structures (Fig. 18).

SUMMARY

Although conventional radiography is still the first diagnostic imaging approach to respiratory disease, CT is proving to be invaluable as an adjunctive procedure in characterizing nasal and thoracic pathologic findings. CT eliminates superimposition of overlying structures and offers superior contrast resolution as compared with conventional radiography. These advantages

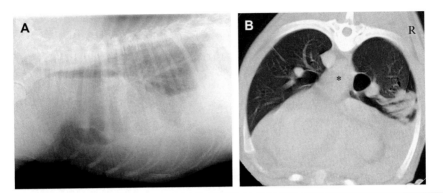

Fig. 18. (A) Right lateral radiograph of a 1-year-old Labrador Retriever with a history of decreased appetite and mild respiratory distress reveals marked pleural effusion with rounding of the lung margins suggestive of chronic inflammatory pleural effusion. Alveolar infiltrates in the left cranial lung lobe may represent atelectasis or bronchopneumonia. (B) CT examination of the same patient reveals loculated pleural and mediastinal fluid accumulation with ill-defined alveolar pulmonary infiltrates in the right middle lung lobe (arrow). Hilar lymphadenopathy is present between the mainstem bronchi (*). Histopathologic examination revealed marked chronic pyogranulomatous mediastinitis and chronic pyogranulomatous pneumonia within the right middle lung lobe. Both regions contained intralesional fungal spherules of Coccidioides immitis.

allow for more precise characterization and localization of lesions and are invaluable for guiding rhinoscopic, bronchoscopic, and surgical procedures.

References

[1] Suter PF. Thoracic radiography a text atlas of thoracic diseases of the dog and cat. Wettswil (Switzerland): P.F. Suter; 1984.

[2] Saunders JH, Van Bree H, Gielen I, et al. Diagnostic value of computed tomography in dogs with chronic nasal disease. Vet Radiol Ultrasound 2003;44(4):409–13.

[3] Sullivan M, Lee R, Jakovljevic S, et al. The radiological features of aspergillosis of the nasal cavity and frontal sinuses in the dog. J Small Anim Pract 1986;27:167–80.

[4] Saunders JH, Zonderland JL, Clercx C, et al. Computed tomographic findings in 35 dogs with nasal aspergillosis. Vet Radiol Ultrasound 2002;43(1):5–9.

[5] Saunders JH, Van Bree H. Comparison of radiography and computed tomography for the diagnosis of canine nasal aspergillosis. Vet Radiol Ultrasound 2003;44(4):414–9.

[6] Wilkinson GT. Feline cryptococcosis: a review and seven case reports. J Small Anim Pract 1979;20:749.

[7] Tomsa K, Glaus TM, Zimmer C, et al. Fungal rhinitis and sinusitis in three cats. J Am Vet Med Assoc 2003;222(10):1380–4.

[8] Harvey CE, Biery DN, Morello J, et al. Chronic nasal disease in the dog: its radiographic diagnosis. Veterinary Radiology 1979;20:91–8.

[9] Schwartz T. Comparison of sensitivity and specificity of conventional radiography and computed tomography (CT) in nasal tumors and fungal rhinitis in dogs. Vet Radiol Ultrasound 1995;36:428.

[10] Burk RL. Computed tomographic imaging of nasal disease in 100 dogs. Vet Radiol Ultrasound 1992;33(3):177–80.

[11] Madewell BR, Priester WA, Gillette EL, et al. Neoplasms of the nasal passages and paranasal sinuses in domesticated animals as reported by 13 veterinary colleges. Am J Vet Res 1976;37:851–6.

[12] Schoenborn WC, Wisner ER, Kass PH, et al. Retrospective assessment of computed tomographic imaging of feline sinonasal disease in 62 cats. Vet Radiol Ultrasound 2003;44(2):185–95.

[13] O'Brien RT, Evans SM, Wortman JA, et al. Radiographic findings in cats with intranasal neoplasia or chronic rhinitis: 29 cases (1982–1988). J Am Vet Med Assoc 1996;208(3):385–9.

[14] Rebner M, Gross BH, Robertson JM, et al. CT evaluation of mediastinal masses. Comput Radiol 1987;11:103–10.

[15] Prather AB, Berry CR, Thrall DE. Use of radiography in combination with computed tomography for the assessment of noncardiac thoracic disease in the dog and cat. Vet Radiol Ultrasound 2005;46(2):114–21.

[16] Bilbrey SA, Birchard SJ. Pulmonary lymphatics in dogs with experimentally induced chylothorax. J Am Anim Hosp Assoc 1994;30:86–91.

[17] Esterline ML, Radlinsky MG, Biller DS, et al. Comparison of radiographic and computed tomography lymphangiography for identification of the canine thoracic duct. Vet Radiol Ultrasound 2005;46(5):391–5.

[18] Johnson EG, Wisner ER, Marks SL, et al. Contrast enhanced CT thoracic duct lymphography. Paper presented at: the annual conference of the American college of veterinary radiology. Chicago: 2006.

[19] Lipscomb VJ, Hardie RJ, Dubielzig RR. Spontaneous pneumothorax caused by pulmonary blebs and bullae in 12 dogs. J Am Anim Hosp Assoc 2003;39:435–45.

[20] Puerto DA, Brockman DJ, Lindquist C, et al. Surgical and nonsurgical management of and selected risk factors for spontaneous pneumothorax in dogs: 64 cases (1986–1999). J Am Vet Med Assoc 2002;220:1670–4.

[21] Au JJ, Weisman DL, Stefanacci JD, et al. Use of computed tomography for evaluation of lung lesions associated with spontaneous pneumothorax in dogs: 12 cases (1999–2002). J Am Vet Med Assoc 2006;228(5):733–7.

[22] Wheeldon EB, Pirie HM, Fisher EW. Chronic bronchitis in the dog. Vet Rec 1974;94:466–71.

[23] Reif JS, Rhodes WH. The lungs of dogs: a radiographic-morphologic correlation. Journal of the American Veterinary Radiologic Society 1966;7:5–11.

[24] Mantis P, Lamb CR, Boswood A. Assessment of the accuracy of thoracic radiography in the diagnosis of canine chronic bronchitis. J Small Anim Pract 1998;39:518–20.

[25] Muller NL, Stales CA, Miller RR, et al. Fibrosing alveolitis: CT-pathologic correlation. Radiology 1986;160:585–8.

[26] Webb WR. High-resolution lung computed tomography. Normal anatomic and pathologic findings. Radiol Clin North Am 1991;29:1058–63.

[27] Spann DR, Sellon RK, Thrall DE, et al. Computed tomographic diagnosis: use of computed tomography to distinguish a pulmonary mass from alveolar disease. Vet Radiol Ultrasound 1998;39(6):532–5.

[28] Berman CG, Clark RA. Diagnostic imaging in cancer. Prim Care 1992;19(4):677–713.

[29] Nemanic S, London CA, Wisner ER. Comparison of thoracic radiographs and single breathhold helical CT for detection of pulmonary nodule in dogs with metastatic neoplasia. J Vet Intern Med 2006;20(3):508–15.

[30] Lobetti RG, Milner RR, Muller NL. Chronic idiopathic pulmonary fibrosis in five dogs. J Am Anim Hosp Assoc 2001;37:119–27.

[31] Corcoran BM, Dukes-McEwan J, Rhind S, et al. Idiopathic pulmonary fibrosis in a Staffordshire bull terrier with hypothyroidism. J Small Anim Pract 1999;40:185–8.

[32] Johnson V, Corcoran BM, Wotton PR, et al. Thoracic high-resolution computed tomographic findings in dogs with canine idiopathic pulmonary fibrosis. J Small Anim Pract 2005;46:381–8.

[33] Leung AN, Miller RR, Muller NL. Parenchymal opacification in chronic infiltrative lung diseases: CT-pathologic correlation. Radiology 1993;188:209–14.

[34] Westcott JL, Cole SR. Traction bronchiectasis in end-stage pulmonary fibrosis. Radiology 1986;161(3):665–9.

Update on Canine Sinonasal Aspergillosis

Dominique Peeters, DVM, PhD*, Cécile Clercx, DVM, PhD

Department of Veterinary Clinical Sciences, Small Animal Internal Medicine,
University of Liège, 20 Boulevard de Colonster B44, 4000 Liège, Belgium

S inonasal aspergillosis (SNA) is the second most common cause of nasal discharge in dogs after nasal neoplasia [1]. The disease is most often caused by *Aspergillus fumigatus*, although occasional cases are caused by other *Aspergillus* species, such as *Aspergillus flavus* or *Aspergillus niger* [2]. Although some suggest that fungi of the genus *Penicillium* cause fungal rhinitis in the dog [2,3], the authors have not observed this. The term *nasal aspergillosis*, which has been used to describe this condition, is better replaced by the term *sinonasal aspergillosis*, because the infection involves the nasal cavity and frontal sinus in most cases [4,5].

PATHOGENESIS

A fumigatus is a filamentous saprophyte and a ubiquitous fungus [6]. In human beings, this organism causes severe disease in immunocompromised individuals or in those with hematologic malignancy [7]. In these patients, *A fumigatus* causes invasive fungal rhinosinusitis, bronchopulmonary aspergillosis, and disseminated aspergillosis [6]. *A fumigatus* is also the primary agent responsible for fungal sinusitis in immune-competent patients [8,9]. Three types of fungal sinusitis occur in immunocompetent patients: allergic fungal sinusitis, fungal ball or mycetoma, and chronic erosive noninvasive fungal sinusitis [8].

In dogs, systemic or disseminated aspergillosis is rare and occurs primarily in German Shepherd Dogs [10,11] or occasionally in other breeds. Affected dogs do not generally have clinical nasal involvement. *Aspergillus terreus* (rather than *A fumigatus*) is the primary causative agent of this condition, for which a systemic immune deficiency is suspected [11,12].

Most dogs with SNA are not systemically immunocompromised [2]; do not have diabetes mellitus, hyperadrenocorticism, or severe leukopenia [13]; and fungal infection is restricted to the nose or frontal sinus [2]. Although impaired peripheral blood lymphocyte proliferative responses have been shown in dogs with SNA [2,14], the significance of this finding is unclear, because *A fumigatus* has been demonstrated to inhibit lymphocyte proliferation in vitro [15].

*Corresponding author. E-mail address: dpeeters@ulg.ac.be (D. Peeters).

0195-5616/07/$ – see front matter
doi:10.1016/j.cvsm.2007.05.005

The absence of systemic immune suppression in dogs with SNA is also suggested by the lack of invasiveness of respiratory mucosa by the fungus [16]. In Grocott-stained sections obtained from nasal biopsies of 15 dogs with SNA, fungal hyphae were seen in only six cases and were not identified within or beneath the mucosal epithelium in any case [16]. In addition, examination of Grocott-stained sections from the frontal bone of 5 dogs with SNA with frontal bone osteomyelitis did not contain fungal elements in bony tissue (M.J. Day, Dominique Peters, DVM, PhD, Cécile Clercx, DVM, PhD, unpublished data, 2004), supporting a lack of fungal tissue invasion. This mimics the situation in people with fungal sinusitis, in which immune-competent patients have noninvasive disease [8].

Despite the fact that SNA is a noninvasive disease in dogs, marked destruction of nasal turbinates is present in all cases [5]. In the most severe cases, there is extensive erosion through frontal bones, through nasal bones into periorbital soft tissue, or through the cribriform plate into the brain [17,18]. Bony destruction is not caused by the fungus itself [16] but is thought to be attributable to the host inflammatory response and to dermonecrolytic fungal toxins [19].

The inflammatory infiltrate found in the nasal or sinusal mucosa of dogs with SNA is dominated by lymphocytes and plasma cells, although neutrophils are present in great numbers in some cases [16]. Eosinophils and mast cells are only rarely observed [16]. The nature of the inflammatory infiltrate can be explained by the chemokine profile found in nasal tissue of dogs with SNA. Upregulation of mRNA encoding interleukin (IL)-8 and monocyte chemoattractant protein (MCP)-1, MCP-2, MCP-3, and MCP-4 is found in the nasal mucosa of dogs with SNA compared with control animals [13]. IL-8 is the primary neutrophil chemoattractant [20], and MCPs attract mostly mononuclear cells [21]. Taken together, the nature of the inflammatory infiltrate, the lack of mucosal invasiveness, the clinical course of the disease, the erosion of bony structures, and the apparent immune competence of affected dogs suggest that canine SNA most resembles the chronic erosive noninvasive fungal sinusitis described in human patients [16].

Aspergillus is a ubiquitous fungus and the reason why *A fumigatus* causes disease in only a small proportion of exposed dogs remains unclear. Many potential virulence factors for *A fumigatus* have been studied in vitro [22]. For example, gliotoxin, aflatoxins, and ribotoxins may interfere with mucociliary clearance, opsonization, and neutrophilic phagocytosis [22–25]. Whether these play a role in canine SNA remains to be determined.

Local immune dysfunction is suspected to be involved in the pathogenesis of canine SNA. Generation of a dominant T helper (Th) 1-cell response, characterized by the activation of CD4+ Th1 cells to produce interferon (IFN)-γ and of macrophages to produce proinflammatory cytokines (eg, IL-6, IL-12, IL-18, and tumor necrosis factor [TNF]-α), is required for the expression of protective acquired immunity to fungi [26]. Cytokine analysis has confirmed that the nasal mucosa of dogs with SNA is dominated by a Th1 response, with upregulation of mRNA encoding IFN-γ, IL-6, IL-12p35, IL-12p40, IL-18, and

TNF-α [13,27]. This strong Th1 and proinflammatory immune response may help to confine *Aspergillus* infection to the nasal cavities and frontal sinuses [27].

mRNA encoding the immunomodulatory cytokine IL-10 is also upregulated in nasal tissue from dogs with SNA [13,27]. The increase in IL-10 transcripts could be implicated in the failure to clear the *Aspergillus* infection from the nose despite a strong mucosal Th1 immune response [13]. Indeed, IL-10 exerts detrimental effects on host responses to fungi [26]. High-level production of IL-10 in the nasal mucosa of dogs with SNA might prove beneficial, however, by limiting the inflammatory response that would lead to extension of local tissue damage initiated by fungal infection [13]. The cause of the increase in IL-10 mRNA expression in dogs with SNA is currently unknown.

In rare cases of canine SNA, a predisposing factor, such as facial trauma, a nasal foreign body, nasal carcinoma, or an impacted tooth, is present [2,19]. These predisposing conditions are thought to alter the nasal epithelium, mucosal resistance, and mucociliary clearance [19].

SIGNALMENT

Although no clear breed predisposition has been reported, SNA affects mainly dogs of mesaticephalic and dolichocephalic breeds [5,16]. Most affected dogs are young adult to middle-aged animals (usually between 1 and 7 years of age), but the disease has been reported in dogs younger than 1 year of age and in old patients [2]. A male predisposition has been observed in several studies [2,4,5].

CLINICAL SIGNS

Typical clinical signs of SNA are profuse mucopurulent to purulent nasal discharge, nasal pain, and ulceration or depigmentation of the nostril [2,5]. This latter sign is almost exclusively seen in SNA and is thought to be caused by fungal toxins in the nasal discharge [28]. The disease usually begins with unilateral mucoid to mucopurulent nasal discharge and can progress to bilateral discharge [2]. Other clinical signs that are often observed are sneezing, reverse sneezing, epistaxis, depression, and decreased appetite [5]. Physical examination often reveals increased nasal air flow. In advanced cases, facial deformity attributable to frontal bone hyperostosis; epiphora secondary to extension of the pathologic process into the orbit; or signs of forebrain dysfunction, such as seizures or dullness, as a result of destruction of the cribriform plate are seen [3,19].

DIAGNOSIS

The diagnosis of SNA is often suspected based on history and clinical findings. Other nasal diseases, such as nasal neoplasia, idiopathic lymphoplasmacytic rhinitis, a nasal foreign body, and oronasal fistula or tooth root abscess, share some clinical features with SNA, however, and a definitive diagnosis is needed before treatment is instituted. Various combinations of diagnostic tests, including radiography, CT, rhinoscopy, sinuscopy, histologic examination, cytology, fungal culture, and serology, are used to confirm the diagnosis of canine SNA [2,4,5,29,30]. Fungal DNA detection is a diagnostic tool that is used in the diagnosis of invasive aspergillosis in human beings [31], but the usefulness of this test in the diagnosis of canine SNA has not been assessed. Currently, no single test can be used to make the diagnosis, because false-positive and false-negative results can occur [30]. To date, the "gold standard" for diagnosing canine SNA is the direct visualization of fungal plaques by rhinoscopy or sinuscopy or the observation of fungal elements on cytology or histopathologic examination of a nasal or sinusal mucosal biopsy [4,5,13,30].

Diagnostic Imaging
Imaging studies should precede rhinoscopy and biopsy procedures to avoid resultant hemorrhage that can obscure subtle imaging lesions and result in focal areas of increased opacity. General anesthesia is required to obtain optimal positioning.

Radiographs of the nasal cavity and frontal sinus have proven useful in the diagnosis of chronic nasal diseases in dogs [32–34]. A typical radiographic finding in SNA is increased radiolucency in the rostral nasal cavity in conjunction with increased radiodensity in the distal aspect [33]. Increased radiodensity is often found in the frontal sinus also [33]. In rare cases, radiographs of the nasal cavities allow the visualization of a nasal foreign body or the detection of dental anomaly that can be associated with SNA [34,35].

CT is becoming more available in veterinary medicine and is widely used for examination of nasal cavity disorders [36,37]. CT offers several advantages relative to conventional radiography for examination of the nasal cavities and frontal sinuses, including cross-sectional imaging that eliminates superimposition of structures, adjustment of the contrast scale to optimize optical density and discriminate fine turbinate structures, and multiplanar reconstructions for better evaluation of the cribriform plate [36,38]. In two recent studies, abnormalities of the nasal cavities were present on CT in all cases with SNA and frontal sinus abnormalities were found in 72% to 74% of the cases [4,18]. The most common CT findings were (1) moderate to severe cavitary destruction of the turbinates, with a variable amount of abnormal soft tissue in the nasal cavities; (2) a rim of soft tissue along the frontal bone, maxillary recess, and nasal bones; (3) and thickened reactive maxillary, vomer, or frontal bone (Fig. 1) [18]. The sensitivity of CT in the diagnosis of SNA is higher than that of radiography [29], particularly in demonstrating the rim of soft tissue along the nasal and frontal bones, frontal bone lesions, and a cavitated process [29]. Moreover, CT can demonstrate cribriform plate lysis that is not visible on radiography [29], which may influence the choice of therapy [39].

MR imaging is also superior to radiography for diagnosing SNA [35]. CT demonstrates bony changes better, however, and there is no clear advantage of using MR imaging in place of CT for the diagnosis of canine SNA [35].

Rhinoscopy or Sinuscopy
Rhinoscopy is considered by many to be the most useful diagnostic tool for canine SNA. In most cases, it allows the visualization of fungal plaques (Fig. 2A)

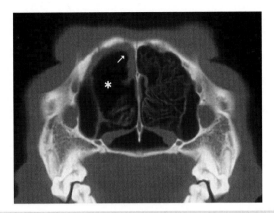

Fig. 1. Transverse CT image of the nasal cavities from a dog with SNA reveals severe turbinate lysis (*) and a rim of soft tissue (*arrow*) in the left nasal cavity. (*Adapted from* Saunders JH, Zonderland JL, Clercx C, et al. Computed tomographic findings in 35 dogs with nasal aspergillosis. Vet Radiol Ultrasound 2002;43:7; with permission.)

[4,5,35] and provides the best method to obtain meaningful samples for mycologic examination by cytology, histopathology, or culture [30]. Moreover, it allows endoscopically guided debridement of affected nasal tissue, which is an essential component of treatment.

Rhinoscopy is performed under general anesthesia. Both nasal cavities are explored using a rigid endoscope with an optical angulation of 0° or 30°. Typical rhinoscopic findings include moderate to severe destruction of turbinates, intranasal mucopurulent secretions, intranasal fungal plaques, and roughening of the mucosa in most cases [5,35]. Nasal septum destruction is observed less frequently (see Fig. 2B) [5,35]. In most cases of aspergillosis with destructive rhinitis and frontal sinus involvement, the frontal sinus(es) can be explored by an experienced endoscopist through the use of antegrade sinuscopy using a flexible

A **B**

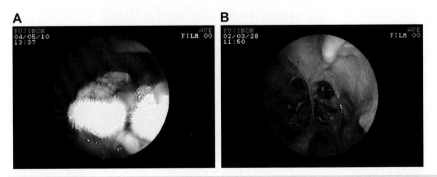

Fig. 2. (*A*) Typical fungal plaque observed during rhinoscopy in a dog with SNA. (*B*) "After cure" rhinoscopic view of the distal part of the nasal cavities in a dog with SNA shows extensive nasal septum lysis.

endoscope [5,35]. Fungal plaques appear as off-white or greenish fuzzy plaques that are adherent to the mucosa. These fungal colonies may rarely be mistaken for mucopurulent exudate by an inexperienced observer [40].

In rare cases, fungal plaques are not observed in the nasal cavity and are seen only in the frontal sinus after sinus trephination and sinuscopy [4]. The authors recommend sinus trephination and sinuscopy for diagnostic purposes only when frontal sinus involvement is confirmed by CT or MRI but rostral rhinoscopy, cytology, or histopathologic examination fails to confirm the diagnosis.

Histopathologic Examination

Histopathologic examination can provide direct evidence of fungal hyphae and a definitive diagnosis of SNA (Fig. 3). Although the specificity of this diagnostic test approximates 100%, the sensitivity depends on the type of biopsy specimen obtained. Sensitivity is quite high when fungal plaques are directly sampled [4], but when adjacent nasal mucosa is sampled, fungal elements are rarely observed [4,16]. This may be a reflection of the lack of mucosal invasion by the fungus [16].

Cytology

Cytologic examination can be helpful in confirming the diagnosis of SNA, and the sensitivity depends on the type of specimen collected [30]. In a study of 15 dogs with SNA, four different sampling methods were compared [30]. Using a direct smear from nasal exudate, fungal hyphae were seen in 13% of the cases and no fungal spores were observed. A blind endonasal swab demonstrated fungal hyphae in 20% of the cases and fungal spores in 7%. Endonasal brushing under endoscopic guidance identified fungal hyphae in 93% of cases, and fungal spores were seen in 27%. A squash preparation of an endonasal biopsy

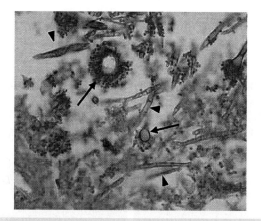

Fig. 3. Histologic examination of a dog shows *Aspergillus* conidia (*arrows*) and hyphae (*arrowheads*) at the surface of the nasal mucosa (periodic acid-Schiff, original magnification ×200). (*From* Saunders JH, van Bree H. Diagnostic modalities of canine nasal aspergillosis. Vlaams Diergeneeskundig Tijdschrift 2003;72:406; with permission.)

obtained with endoscopic guidance showed fungal hyphae in 100% of cases and fungal spores in 33% [30]. Thus, the sensitivity of cytology in the diagnosis of SNA is high if the sample is collected directly from fungal plaques, but the diagnostic value of cytology is poor when fungal plaques are not visualized and sampled.

Fungal Culture

Fungal culture has long been considered of little value in the diagnosis of canine SNA [2], likely because culture of nasal discharge leads to a high number of false-negative results [2,41]. When mucosal biopsies or fungal plaque samples are submitted for culture, the sensitivity of fungal culture in the diagnosis of SNA increases to between 40% and 77% [4,5,42]. Culture of nasal discharge has been reported to yield positive results in 30% to 40% of cases in normal dogs and dogs with neoplasia [2,41], although in the authors' experience and in a recent report [42], positive fungal cultures are rarely obtained in dogs without SNA.

Given the robust growth of *Aspergillus* species in the environment, the poor clinical yield from infected tissue or secretions seems paradoxic. Poor yield of *Aspergillus* spp in culture could be attributable to suboptimal laboratory methodology. Incubating fungal cultures from clinical samples (sputum, bronchial wash, or lavage specimens) from human patients with bronchopulmonary aspergillosis at 35°C instead of 25°C improved recovery of *Aspergillus* spp from 5% to 43% [43]. It is theorized that *Aspergillus* adapts to the physiologic temperature of the host tissue and is unable to grow when transferred to an artificial culture medium kept at ambient temperature [43]. Therefore, laboratory conditions should be investigated before submitting samples for fungal culture.

Serology

Several techniques for determining serum *Aspergillus*-specific antibody titers have been evaluated. Agar gel immunodiffusion (AGID) is widely used because it is inexpensive and easy to perform [6]. The primary disadvantage of this method is an inability to quantify the immune response [6]. In the authors' experience with AGID using the "*Aspergillus fumigatus* immunodiffusion system" (Immuno-Mycologics, Oklahoma), the sensitivity of this method in the diagnosis of SNA is quite low (31%), but false-positive results are only rarely obtained. In a recent study using an AGID test from Merridian Diagnostics (Cincinnati, Ohio), a test using *Aspergillus* antigen from cultures of *A fumigatus, A niger,* and *A flavus,* sensitivity was somewhat higher at 68% and specificity was 98% [42]. The experience of the laboratory personnel reading the test is likely important.

Counterimmunoelectrophoresis can assist with diagnosis of canine SNA [2] but is not in widespread use. ELISA to detect anti-*Aspergillus* antibodies in canine serum is an alternative to AGID [2,44] and provides the benefit of quantitation of the immune response. Nevertheless, the diagnostic value of this method in SNA has not been established.

The detection of *Aspergillus* galactomannan by a sandwich ELISA method is currently used for the early diagnosis of invasive aspergillosis in human beings and is highly sensitive and specific [6]. Because SNA is not an invasive disease in the dog [16], the probability of detecting circulating antigens in serum of affected dogs is likely low. One study investigated serum galactomannan detection in three dogs with nasal aspergillosis, and the result was negative in all cases [44].

Fungal DNA Quantification

In human medicine, the detection of *Aspergillus* DNA in serum or whole blood by real-time polymerase chain reaction is part of the diagnostic investigation in patients at risk for invasive aspergillosis [31]. The usefulness of quantifying whole blood and tissue fungal and *A fumigatus* DNA in the diagnosis of canine SNA is currently under investigation, although preliminary results suggest no advantage of these measurements over serology or fungal culture.

TREATMENT

Effective treatment of SNA in dogs has always been difficult and is still a challenge. Treatments include systemic antifungal therapy, topical antimycotic therapy, and invasive surgical procedures. Reported success rates and outcome vary depending on the method used to establish cure.

Systemic oral treatment with antifungal agents is noninvasive but requires prolonged administration because of poor to moderate efficacy. This method of treatment is quite expensive, and side effects, such as hepatotoxicosis, anorexia, or vomiting, are commonly reported [45]. Drugs used orally include thiabendazole (10 mg/kg administered per os every 12 hours for 6–8 weeks) [46], ketoconazole (5 mg/kg administered per os every 12 hours for 6–18 weeks) [47], itraconazole (5 mg/kg administered per os every 12 hours for 10 weeks) [45], and fluconazole (2.5 mg/kg administered per os every 12 hours for 10 weeks) [17]. Clinical cure is reported in approximately half of the patients treated with thiabendazole and ketoconazole and in as many as 70% of patients treated with itraconazole or fluconazole.

Topical treatment with clotrimazole or enilconazole has been associated with greater success and has improved management of SNA. These drugs have poor solubility and limited intestinal absorption, and are therefore used topically [39,48]. They are fungistatic at low concentrations but fungicidal at higher concentrations [48,49]. Enilconazole, like the other azole derivatives, inhibits sterol synthesis and also inhibits synthesis of nucleic acids, triglycerides, fatty acids, and oxidative enzymes [48,49]. At a high local concentration, clotrimazole causes direct damage to fungal membranes and inhibits fungal ergosterol synthesis [50]. Clotrimazole preparations contain isopropanol and propylene glycol and are irritating to mucous membranes, causing pharyngeal irritation and edema [51]. Enilconazole is less toxic and irritating, especially at low concentrations [48], and may demonstrate antifungal activity in the vapor phase over a distance of 1 cm [52].

When topical therapy of SNA was first introduced, tubes were implanted surgically into the frontal sinus and enilconazole was instilled twice daily for 7 to 14 days. Resolution of nasal discharge was reported in 80% of the dogs [39]. An alternative technique using a single 1-hour infusion of clotrimazole was introduced as a less invasive and time-intensive therapy and resulted in resolution of clinical signs in up to 85% of affected dogs, with almost half of the cases resolving after a single treatment [53]. Clotrimazole was instilled under general anesthesia through catheters placed surgically in the frontal sinus or through endoscopy. This method reduced hospitalization time and eliminated the complications associated with indwelling catheters.

Currently, noninvasive techniques using endoscopically placed catheters are employed most commonly to infuse drug topically into the nasal cavities and frontal sinus. The use of these methods eliminates the need for surgical trephination and is associated with fewer complications [5,53,54]. Several treatment protocols have been investigated to improve the success rate, tolerance by the animal, and owner compliance. Tubes are placed blindly [53] or endoscopically [5,54] into the nasal cavity or the frontal sinus, and enilconazole or clotrimazole is used at various concentrations. Rhinoscopic evaluation for resolution of disease and drug infusion is repeated at 3- to 4-week intervals as needed. These methods show an improved efficacy, reaching a success rate of up to 80% to 90% [5,53,54].

Clotrimazole infusion is performed under general anesthesia while the dog is intubated with a cuffed endotracheal tube (Fig. 4). An early study evaluated the distribution of dye injected into cadaver skulls of normal dogs and demonstrated that a noninvasive technique for intranasal infusion resulted in better distribution of infusate within the nasal cavity and paranasal sinuses than did techniques using catheters placed by means of sinusotomy [55]. Also, in 12 dogs with fungal rhinitis, bilateral administration of 50 mL into each nasal cavity resulted in excellent distribution of infusate to the entire cavity and frontal sinuses, as determined by evaluation of pre- and postinfusion images on CT

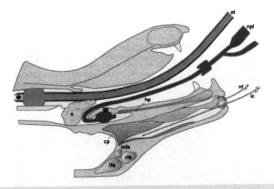

Fig. 4. Sagittal section shows the position of the endotracheal tube (et), nasopharyngeal Foley catheter (npf), pharyngeal sponges (s), infusion catheter (ic), and rostral nasal Foley catheter in relation to the hard palate (hp), soft palate (sp), cribriform plate (cp), rostral frontal sinus (rfs), medial frontal sinus (mfs), and lateral frontal sinus (lfs). (*From* Mathews KG, Davidson AP, Koblik PD, et al. Comparison of topical administration of clotrimazole through surgically placed versus nonsurgically placed catheters for treatment of nasal aspergillosis in dogs: 60 cases (1990–1996). J Am Vet Med Assoc 1998;213(4):503; with permission.)

[37]. Importantly, when tubes were placed correctly, there was minimal leakage into the pharynx [55]. The tip of a 24-French Foley catheter is inserted through the mouth dorsal to the soft palate at the junction between the hard and soft palate, where a 30 mL-balloon is inflated to occlude the nasopharynx. A moistened lap pad is placed in the pharynx to avoid leakage of drugs into the trachea and to help keep the Foley catheter in place. One 10- or 12-French polypropylene drug infusion catheter is advanced dorsomedially in each nostril to the level of the medial canthus of the palpebral fissure. When possible, infusion catheters can be placed under endoscopic guidance with a flexible bronchoscope into the caudal part of the frontal sinus to improve drug delivery (Fig. 5) [54]. A 12-French Foley catheter is then inserted in each nostril, and the balloons are inflated to occlude the nostrils. Additional cotton swabs can be placed in the nostrils to aid in retention of drug within the nasal cavity. Each drug infusion catheter is connected to a 60-mL infusion syringe filled with the topical drug, and constant infusion is performed by use of a syringe driver. When the nasal cavity and frontal sinus are sufficiently filled with drug, leakage from the Foley catheters is noted. At that stage, the catheters should be clamped. The dog's head is rotated every 15 minutes into dorsal recumbency, left lateral recumbency, right lateral recumbency, and ventral recumbency to ensure drug contact with all nasal surfaces.

At the end of the intranasal infusion, the head is tilted downward at an angle of 30°, the lap pad and catheters are removed, and the nasal cavities are allowed to drain for 20 minutes. The pharynx and larynx are examined before the dog is allowed to recover from anesthesia. Complications during the procedure include leakage of drug around the catheters or through accessory incisive ducts of the nasolacrimal system and, rarely, bleeding at withdrawal of catheters [53].

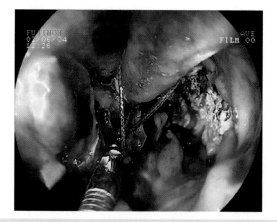

Fig. 5. Perendoscopic placement of a catheter in the frontal sinus for enilconazole topical therapy. A typical fungal plaque is present right to the catheter.

Topical administration of clotrimazole resulted in clinical cure in 65% of dogs after one treatment and in 87% of dogs after two or more treatments [53]. In another study, enilconazole was administered nasally as a 1% solution or into the frontal sinus as a 2% solution and treatment response was evaluated [5]. First, this study confirmed that extensive rhinoscopic debridement before infusion is an important element for therapeutic success. Second, this study demonstrated a success rate of 92% with infusion of 1% or 2% enilconazole emulsion. Third, administration of 2% enilconazole into the frontal sinus by means of endoscopically placed catheters seemed to reduce the number of treatments required for cure. In all dogs, profuse nasal discharge and sneezing were the major adverse effects noted during the immediate posttreatment period [5], but these improved markedly within 24 hours. None of the dogs had anesthetic or neurologic complications. Final follow-up rhinoscopy in all dogs revealed the absence of fungal plaques and the presence of mucosal blebs resulting from the treatment procedure (Fig. 6) [5]. Rare complications of this technique might include partial occlusion of the nare(s) or at the entrance to the frontal sinus (Fig. 7) as a result of the formation of scar tissue from severe ulceration and inflammation. Chronic obstructive sinusitis might be a sequel to antifungal treatment.

Rhinoscopy is useful for topical treatment and is recommended to assess short-term cure [5,54]. Few studies have addressed the long-term outcome in dogs with SNA [39,53,56]. In two studies of dogs treated with clotrimazole or enilconazole, no permanent nasal signs were reported 5 to 61 months after treatment, although antibiotic-responsive nasal discharge occurred in 7 of 57 dogs and 5 of 31 dogs, respectively [39,53]. In a more recent study of 27 dogs with SNA treated with topical enilconazole, approximately half of the dogs showed mild episodic or permanent nasal signs 5 to 64 months after treatment, which were thought to result from extensive turbinate destruction

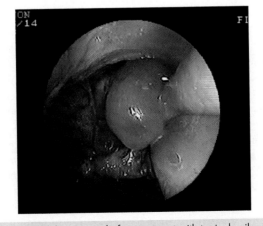

Fig. 6. Typical mucosal bleb appeared after treatment with topical enilconazole in the nasal cavity of a dog with SNA.

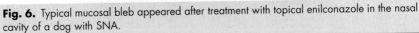

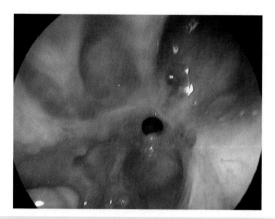

Fig. 7. Severe fibrous reaction occurred at the entrance of the frontal sinus after topical therapy with enilconazole.

[56]. Three dogs demonstrated clinical recurrence of SNA 2, 23, and 36 months after cure, respectively. Among these dogs, cure had been established by means of follow-up rhinoscopy, and they had been all been asymptomatic until relapse [56]. This shows that recurrence of SNA, although not frequent, is possible.

Topical infusion of clotrimazole or enilconazole might be contraindicated in dogs with CT evidence of damage to the cribriform plate, although it has been completed in some dogs without complications and with therapeutic success [5]. Potential complications to be aware of in dogs with evidence of cribriform destruction include development of neurologic signs compatible with cortical encephalopathy or meningitis. Ideally, CT should be performed before each treatment to assess the integrity of the cribriform plate, although this is not always possible financially.

Use of topical agents by means of the noninvasive technique is well tolerated and results in a high success rate; however, these procedures are time-consuming and require prolonged anesthetic time. In a recent study, clotrimazole cream was instilled into the frontal sinus after trephination to act as a depot agent for extended drug contact and minimization of anesthetic time [57]. Fourteen dogs were treated by frontal sinus trephination and a short 5-minute flushing of 1% topical clotrimazole solution followed by 1% clotrimazole cream. Treatment was well tolerated by all patients; 12 (86%) of 14 dogs responded well to treatment and had no clinical signs 6 months after treatment or signs consistent with mild rhinitis [57]. Only 1 dog required multiple treatments.

Despite all efforts, some dogs remain refractory to any treatment, and the prognosis for these patients is poor. Therefore, there is still room for more invasive surgical procedures in selected poorly responsive dogs. Three dogs with refractory mycotic rhinitis were treated by use of temporary rhinostomy and topical povidone-iodine dressings to produce sustained release of povidone-iodine [58]. This treatment was designed because there is some evidence that topical povidone-iodine used as a "paint" after open rhinotomy can be considered an alternative treatment for SNA [59]. The use of a slow-release form of dressing was expected to maintain adequate levels of active iodine locally and to reduce the frequency of handling the animal. Although successful, the topical povidone-iodine pack used in this study was more invasive than any other alternative option, which makes it unsuitable for routine use.

Another surgical method described in seven dogs with severe or recurrent SNA used rhinotomy and surgical debridement associated with topical administration of 2% enilconazole [60]. Rhinotomy with removal of the bone flap and infusion of 2% enilconazole over 1 hour resulted in a satisfactory outcome; however, when the bone flap was not removed, persistence of fungal colonies was noted on the flap or at the level of a cerclage wire closure in 100% of cases.

SUMMARY

Canine SNA is most commonly caused by *A fumigatus*. Local immune dysfunction is suspected in affected dogs, and increased local expression of IL-10 may play a central role in the pathogenesis of the disease. Although clinical signs are quite typical, definitive diagnosis can be difficult to achieve. CT and MRI are useful for evaluating the extent of disease, and the gold standard for diagnosing disease is direct visualization of fungal plaques by endoscopy or the observation of fungal elements on cytology or histopathologic examination. Topical treatment with clotrimazole or enilconazole using minimally invasive techniques is associated with a high success rate and few complications in most cases. Multiple treatments are often required, however. Extensive debridement of fungal plaques is essential to allow contact of the topical drug, and follow-up rhinoscopy aids in assessing response to treatment.

References

[1] Windsor RC, Johnson LR, Herrgesell EJ, et al. Idiopathic lymphoplasmacytic rhinitis in dogs: 37 cases (1997–2002). J Am Vet Med Assoc 2004;224(12):1952–7.

[2] Sharp NJH, Harvey CE, Sullivan M. Canine nasal aspergillosis and penicilliosis. Compendium on Continuing Education for the Practicing Veterinarian 1991;13:41–7.

[3] Mathews K. Fungal rhinitis. In: King L, editor. Textbook of respiratory disease in dogs and cats. St Louis (MO): Saunders; 2004. p. 284–93.

[4] Johnson LR, Drazenovich TL, Herrera MA, et al. Results of rhinoscopy alone or in conjunction with sinuscopy in dogs with aspergillosis: 46 cases (2001–2004). J Am Vet Med Assoc 2006;228(5):738–42.

[5] Zonderland JL, Stork CK, Saunders JH, et al. Intranasal infusion of enilconazole for treatment of sinonasal aspergillosis in dogs. J Am Vet Med Assoc 2002;221(10):1421–5.

[6] Latge JP. *Aspergillus fumigatus* and aspergillosis. Clin Microbiol Rev 1999;12(2):310–50.

[7] Hasan RA, Abuhammour W. Invasive aspergillosis in children with hematologic malignancies. Paediatr Drugs 2006;8(1):15–24.

[8] Uri N, Cohen-Kerem R, Elmalah I, et al. Classification of fungal sinusitis in immunocompetent patients. Otolaryngol Head Neck Surg 2003;129(4):372–8.

[9] Hamilos DL, Lund VJ. Etiology of chronic rhinosinusitis: the role of fungus. Ann Otol Rhinol Laryngol Suppl 2004;193:27–31.

[10] Clercx C, McEntee K, Snaps F, et al. Bronchopulmonary and disseminated granulomatous disease associated with *Aspergillus fumigatus* and *Candida* species infection in a golden retriever. J Am Anim Hosp Assoc 1996;32(2):139–45.

[11] Day MJ, Penhale WJ. An immunohistochemical study of canine disseminated aspergillosis. Aust Vet J 1991;68(12):383–6.

[12] Day MJ, Eger CE, Shaw SE, et al. Immunologic study of systemic aspergillosis in German shepherd dogs. Vet Immunol Immunopathol 1985;9(4):335–47.

[13] Peeters D, Peters IR, Clercx C, et al. Quantification of mRNA encoding cytokines and chemokines in nasal biopsies from dogs with sino-nasal aspergillosis. Vet Microbiol 2006; 114(3–4):318–26.

[14] Barrett RE, Hoffer RE, Schultz RD. Treatment and immunological evaluation of 3 cases of canine aspergillosis. J Am Anim Hosp Assoc 1977;13:328–34.

[15] Chaparas SD, Morgan PA, Holobaugh P, et al. Inhibition of cellular immunity by products of *Aspergillus fumigatus*. J Med Vet Mycol 1986;24(1):67–76.

[16] Peeters D, Day MJ, Clercx C. An immunohistochemical study of canine nasal aspergillosis. J Comp Pathol 2005;132(4):283–8.

[17] Sharp NJH, Harvey CE, Obrien JA. Treatment of canine nasal aspergillosis penicilliosis with fluconazole (UK-49,858). J Small Anim Pract 1991;32(10):513–6.

[18] Saunders JH, Zonderland JL, Clercx C, et al. Computed tomographic findings in 35 dogs with nasal aspergillosis. Vet Radiol Ultrasound 2002;43(1):5–9.

[19] Saunders JH, van Bree H. Diagnostic modalities of canine nasal aspergillosis. Vlaams Diergeneeskundig Tijdschrift 2003;72:399–408.

[20] Kunkel SL, Standiford T, Kasahara K, et al. Interleukin-8 (IL-8): the major neutrophil chemotactic factor in the lung. Exp Lung Res 1991;17(1):17–23.

[21] Lloyd C. Chemokines in allergic lung inflammation. Immunology 2002;105(2):144–54.

[22] Tomee JF, Kauffman HF. Putative virulence factors of *Aspergillus fumigatus*. Clin Exp Allergy 2000;30(4):476–84.

[23] Amitani R, Taylor G, Elezis EN, et al. Purification and characterization of factors produced by *Aspergillus fumigatus* which affect human ciliated respiratory epithelium. Infect Immun 1995;63(9):3266–71.

[24] Cusumano V, Costa GB, Seminara S. Effect of aflatoxins on rat peritoneal macrophages. Appl Environ Microbiol 1990;56(11):3482–4.

[25] Eichner RD, Al Salami M, Wood PR, et al. The effect of gliotoxin upon macrophage function. Int J Immunopharmacol 1986;8(7):789–97.

[26] Romani L. Immunity to fungal infections. Nat Rev Immunol 2004;4(1):1–23.

[27] Peeters D, Peters IR, Helps CR, et al. Distinct tissue cytokine and chemokine mRNA expression in canine sino-nasal aspergillosis and idiopathic lymphoplasmacytic rhinitis. Vet Immunol Immunopathol 2007;117(1-2):95–105.

[28] Sharp NJH, Sullivan M, Harvey CE. Treatment of canine nasal aspergillosis. In Pract 1992;14:27–31.

[29] Saunders JH, van Bree H. Comparison of radiography and computed tomography for the diagnosis of canine nasal aspergillosis. Vet Radiol Ultrasound 2003;44(4):414–9.

[30] De Lorenzi D, Bonfanti U, Masserdotti C, et al. Diagnosis of canine nasal aspergillosis by cytological examination: a comparison of four different collection techniques. J Small Anim Pract 2006;47(6):316–9.

[31] Ferns RB. Evaluation of the role of real-time PCR in the diagnosis of invasive aspergillosis. Leuk Lymphoma 2006;47(1):15–20.

[32] Sullivan M, Lee R, Skae CA. The radiological features of 60 cases of intranasal neoplasia in the dog. J Small Anim Pract 1987;28(7):575–86.

[33] Sullivan M, Lee R, Jakovljevic S, et al. The radiological features of aspergillosis of the nasal cavity and frontal sinuses in the dog. J Small Anim Pract 1986;27:167–80.

[34] Gibbs C, Lane JG, Denny HR. Radiological features of intra-nasal lesions in the dog: a review of 100 cases. J Small Anim Pract 1979;20(9):515–35.

[35] Saunders JH, Clercx C, Snaps FR, et al. Radiographic, magnetic resonance imaging, computed tomographic, and rhinoscopic features of nasal aspergillosis in dogs. J Am Vet Med Assoc 2004;225(11):1703–12.

[36] Burk RL. Computed tomographic imaging of nasal disease in 100 dogs. Vet Radiol Ultrasound 1992;33(3):177–80.

[37] Mathews KG, Koblik PD, Richardson EF, et al. Computed tomographic assessment of noninvasive intranasal infusions in dogs with fungal rhinitis. Vet Surg 1996;25(4):309–19.

[38] Codner EC, Lurus AG, Miller JB, et al. Comparison of computed tomography with radiography as a noninvasive diagnostic technique for chronic nasal disease in dogs. J Am Vet Med Assoc 1993;202(7):1106–10.

[39] Sharp NJH, Sullivan M, Harvey CE, et al. Treatment of canine nasal aspergillosis with enilconazole. J Vet Intern Med 1993;7(1):40–3.

[40] McCarthy TC, McDermaid SL. Rhinoscopy. Vet Clin North Am Small Anim Pract 1990; 20(5):1265–90.

[41] Harvey CE, O'Brien JA, Felsburg PJ, et al. Nasal penicilliosis in six dogs. J Am Vet Med Assoc 1981;178(10):1084–7.

[42] Pomrantz JS, Johnson LR, Nelson RW, et al. Comparison of serologic evaluation via agar gel immunodiffusion and fungal culture of tissue for diagnosis of nasal aspergillosis in dogs. J Am Vet Med Assoc 2007;230(9):1319–23.

[43] Tarrand JJ, Han XY, Kontoyiannis DP, et al. *Aspergillus* hyphae in infected tissue: evidence of physiologic adaptation and effect on culture recovery. J Clin Microbiol 2005;43(1): 382–6.

[44] Garcia ME, Caballero J, Cruzado M, et al. The value of the determination of anti-*Aspergillus* IgG in the serodiagnosis of canine aspergillosis: comparison with galactomannan detection. J Vet Med B Infect Dis Vet Public Health 2001;48(10):743–50.

[45] Legendre A. Antimycotic drug therapy. In: Bonagura J, editor. Kirk's current veterinary therapy XII. Philadelphia: WB Saunders Co; 1995. p. 327–31.

[46] Harvey CE. Nasal aspergillosis and penicilliosis in dogs: results of treatment with thiabendazole. J Am Vet Med Assoc 1984;184(1):48–50.

[47] Sharp NJ, Sullivan M. Use of ketoconazole in the treatment of canine nasal aspergillosis. J Am Vet Med Assoc 1989;194(6):782–6.

[48] Sharp NJ. Aspergillosis and penicilliosis. In: Greene C, editor. Infectious diseases of the dog and cat. Philadelphia: WB Saunders; 1998. p. 404–13.

[49] McGinnis M, Rinaldi M. Antifungal drugs: mechanisms of action, drug resistance, susceptibility testing, and assays of activity in biologic fluids. In: Lorian V, editor. Antibiotics in laboratory medicine. Baltimore (MD): MA Williams and Wilkins; 1991. p. 176–211.

[50] Iwata K, Yamaguchi H, Hiratani T. Mode of action of clotrimazole. Sabouraudia 1973; 11(2):158–66.

[51] Caulkett N, Lew L, Fries C. Upper-airway obstruction and prolonged recovery from anesthesia following intranasal clotrimazole administration. J Am Anim Hosp Assoc 1997;33(3): 264–7.

[52] Van Gestel J, Van Cutsem J, Thienpont D. Vapour phase activity of imazalil. Chemotherapy 1981;27(4):270–6.

[53] Mathews KG, Davidson AP, Koblik PD, et al. Comparison of topical administration of clotrimazole through surgically placed versus nonsurgically placed catheters for treatment of nasal aspergillosis in dogs: 60 cases (1990–1996). J Am Vet Med Assoc 1998;213(4): 501–6.

[54] McCullough SM, McKiernan BC, Grodsky BS. Endoscopically placed tubes for administration of enilconazole for treatment of nasal aspergillosis in dogs. J Am Vet Med Assoc 1998;212(1):67–9.

[55] Richardson EF, Mathews KG. Distribution of topical agents in the frontal sinuses and nasal cavity of dogs: comparison between current protocols for treatment of nasal aspergillosis and a new noninvasive technique. Vet Surg 1995;24(6):476–83.

[56] Schuller S, Clercx C. Long-term outcomes in dogs with sinonasal aspergillosis treated with intranasal infusions of enilconazole. J Am Anim Hosp Assoc 2007;43(1):33–8.

[57] Sissener TR, Bacon NJ, Friend E, et al. Combined clotrimazole irrigation and depot therapy for canine nasal aspergillosis. J Small Anim Pract 2006;47(6):312–5.

[58] Hotston Moore A. Topical povidone-iodine dressings in the management of mycotic rhinitis in three dogs. J Small Anim Pract 2003;44:326–9.

[59] Pavletic MM, Clark GN. Open nasal cavity and frontal sinus treatment of chronic canine aspergillosis. Vet Surg 1991;20(1):43–8.

[60] Claeys S, Lefebvre JB, Schuller S, et al. Surgical treatment of canine nasal aspergillosis by rhinotomy combined with enilconazole infusion and oral itraconazole. J Small Anim Pract 2006;47(6):320–4.

Canine Eosinophilic Bronchopneumopathy

Cécile Clercx, DVM, PhD*, Dominique Peeters, DVM, PhD

Department of Veterinary Clinical Sciences, Small Animal Internal Medicine, University of Liège, 20 Boulevard de Colonster–B44, 4000 Liège, Belgium

Infiltration of the airways or pulmonary parenchyma by eosinophils has been described in the dog as pulmonary infiltration with eosinophils (PIE) [1], pulmonary eosinophilia (PE) [2], eosinophilic pneumonia [3], and eosinophilic bronchopneumopathy (EBP) [4]; however, to date, no clear method of classification exists. The authors use the term *eosinophilic bronchopneumopathy* rather than *pulmonary infiltration with eosinophils* or *pulmonary eosinophilia*, because EBP takes into account the fact that bronchial infiltration and parenchymal involvement are almost always present in these cases. A cause is rarely identified, and most cases of EBP are considered idiopathic [4].

In human medicine, eosinophilic lower airway diseases are a heterogeneous group of disorders in which an increased number of eosinophils are present in the airways or lung parenchyma [5]. These diseases are broadly separated into airway and parenchymal disorders (Box 1). In some cases, eosinophils are merely a part of the inflammatory process and may even be present to protect host tissues against parasites or other organisms. In other cases, eosinophils seem to be directly responsible for tissue damage [5].

This article presents the classification of eosinophilic lower airway diseases that is commonly used in human medicine (see Box 1) and proposes an adapted classification for the dog (Box 2). This classification is followed by a review of the current understanding of canine idiopathic EBP.

CLASSIFICATION OF EOSINOPHILIC LOWER AIRWAY DISEASES

Airway Disorders

Asthma is the most frequent cause of airway eosinophilia in human beings. This condition is characterized by chronic cough, eosinophilic infiltration of the bronchial wall, reversible air flow obstruction, and bronchial hyperactivity [6]. The syndrome of asthma has not been recognized in dogs, although the authors have observed apparent bronchial hyperactivity in some advanced cases of canine EBP (see section on pulmonary function tests [PFTs]).

*Corresponding author. E-mail address: cclercx@ulg.ac.be (C. Clercx).

0195-5616/07/$ – see front matter
doi:10.1016/j.cvsm.2007.05.007

Box 1: Classification of eosinophilic lower airway disorders in human beings

Airway disorders
Asthma
Eosinophilic bronchitis
Allergic bronchopulmonary aspergillosis
Bronchocentric granulomatosis

Parenchymal disorders associated with known underlying condition
Parasitic infections
Other infections (mycobacteria, fungi)
Interstitial lung diseases
Drug reactions
Idiopathic hypereosinophilic syndrome
Pulmonary vasculitis
Lung cancer
Others

Idiopathic parenchymal disorders
Simple PE
Chronic eosinophilic pneumonia
Acute eosinophilic pneumonia

(*Data from* Alberts WM. Eosinophilic interstitial lung disease. Curr Opin Pulm Med 2004; 10:420.)

Eosinophilic bronchitis (EB) is a condition in human medicine characterized by a corticosteroid-responsive cough, bronchial eosinophilia, no airway obstruction, and normal airway responsiveness [7]. Whether asthma and EB are distinct entities or conditions representing a pathophysiologic spectrum of disease awaits further elucidation [8], but it has been shown that repeated episodes of EB can be associated with the development of asthma in people [9]. Although canine EB has been documented in the veterinary literature [1,10], eosinophilic tracheobronchitis without obvious pulmonary parenchymal involvement has been observed in only a few dogs.

Allergic bronchopulmonary aspergillosis (ABPA) is a rare complication of asthma or cystic fibrosis in human beings [11]. In this disease entity, airway colonization by *Aspergillus* exacerbates underlying asthmatic injury. Pathologic manifestations of ABPA include mucoid impaction of bronchi, bronchocentric granulomatosis, eosinophilic pneumonia, and chronic bronchiolitis [11]. Although *Aspergillus fumigatus* has been cultured from bronchoalveolar fluid (BALF) of two dogs with EBP, fungal hyphae were not observed on cytology

Box 2: Classification of eosinophilic lower airway disorders in dogs

Airway disorders
Idiopathic eosinophilic bronchitis or tracheobronchitis
Parasitic tracheobronchitis (*Oslerus osleri*)

Parenchymal disorders associated with known underlying condition
Parasitic infections
Occult heartworm disease (presenting as eosinophilic pneumonitis or as eosinophilic granulomatous pneumonia)
Angiostrongylus vasorum, Filaroides hirthi
Chronic bacterial pneumonia (aspiration pneumonia, foreign body pneumonia)
Idiopathic hypereosinophilic syndrome
Eosinophilic pulmonary vasculitis?
Lung cancer
Other?

Idiopathic parenchymal disorder
Eosinophilic granulomatous pneumonia
Simple eosinophilic pneumonia?

Idiopathic mixed (airway and parenchyma) disorder
EBP (also referred to in the veterinary literature as PIE or PE)

of BALF or in bronchial biopsies from these dogs [4], and it does not seem that ABPA specifically exists in the dog.

In human beings, bronchocentric granulomatosis is an unusual pathologic entity characterized by granulomatous inflammation affecting the bronchi and bronchioles [12]. The inflammation consists of a dense infiltrate of eosinophils, lymphocytes, and plasma cells surrounded by palisading epithelioid cells; destruction of smaller airways ultimately results. In asthmatic people, bronchocentric granulomatosis is considered to be an immunologic reaction to endobronchial fungi, particularly *A fumigatus*. In nonasthmatic people, evidence for endobronchial infection with *Aspergillus* is usually absent and a causative agent is often not identified [13]. This condition has not yet been reported in dogs.

Parenchymal Disorders Associated with Known Underlying Condition

Several parasites, such as *Strongyloides* spp, *Ascaris* spp, *Toxocara canis*, *Ancylostoma* spp, or *Wuchereria bancrofti*, can lead to eosinophilic pneumonia in human beings. In most of theses parasitic diseases, respiratory symptoms are mild and gastroenterologic signs dominate the clinical picture [5]. In the dog, occult heartworm disease caused by *Dirofilaria immitis* can cause eosinophilic pneumonitis because of antibody-dependent leukocyte adhesion to microfilariae in the pulmonary circulation, entrapment of microfilariae in the capillaries, and subsequent granulomatous inflammation [14]. In some cases, inflammation is dominated by eosinophils [14], whereas in others, granulomatous inflammation progresses to eosinophilic pulmonary granulomatosis, a condition that behaves similar to malignant pulmonary histiocytosis [15].

Migration of larvae of *Angiostrongylus vasorum* through pulmonary parenchyma can result in eosinophilic pneumonia in dogs [16], although in most cases, neutrophils rather than eosinophils predominate in BALF [17]. The primary clinical signs in affected dogs are cough, respiratory difficulty, and hemorrhagic diathesis [17].

Other parasites, such as *Oslerus osleri*, *Filaroides hirthi*, *Crenosema vulpis*, or *Paragonimus kellicotti*, have been implicated in the influx of eosinophils into the airways (*O osleri*) or lungs (other parasites) in dogs [18].

In chronic pulmonary infections caused by mycobacteria or fungi in human beings, eosinophils may comprise a significant proportion of the inflammatory infiltrate [5]. This has also been suggested in the dog [19] but has not been confirmed in the veterinary literature. In the authors' experience, however, pulmonary infection caused by severe aspiration pneumonia or a foreign body can lead to eosinophilic infiltration in chronic cases.

Although an increased eosinophil count is reported in human interstitial lung diseases, such as idiopathic pulmonary fibrosis or sarcoidosis [5], the importance of eosinophils in the pathogenesis of these disorders is uncertain. Idiopathic pulmonary fibrosis in dogs [20] is not associated with eosinophilic infiltrates.

Several drugs have been associated with eosinophilic pneumonia in human beings [21]. Most medications associated with this reaction are antibiotics or nonsteroidal anti-inflammatory drugs [3]. Most cases are isolated, and clinical signs are usually mild and resolve by simply discontinuing the medication [5]. To the authors' knowledge, drug-induced eosinophilic pneumonia has not been reported in dogs.

In humans, idiopathic hypereosinophilic syndrome is a rare illness of unknown cause marked by sustained overproduction of eosinophils and infiltration of multiple organs by mature eosinophils [22]. In dogs, a similar and rare condition is reported, particularly in Rottweilers [23,24]. The disease has to be differentiated from eosinophilic leukemia by bone marrow aspirate [24]. Affected dogs usually display anorexia, depression, and weight loss. Other clinical signs depend on the organs infiltrated by eosinophils and include cough, vomiting, or diarrhea. Some dogs may respond well to prednisolone or hydroxyurea [24,25], although, in general, the prognosis is poor.

In human medicine, eosinophils can be associated with lung lesions that accompany pulmonary vasculitis syndromes. Eosinophilic pulmonary vasculitis is most commonly found in association with primary systemic vasculitis, but primary pulmonary vasculitis, such as Churg-Strauss syndrome, is also reported [5]. Currently, there is no peer-reviewed report in the veterinary literature describing eosinophilic pulmonary vasculitis in the dog, although eosinophilic pulmonary vasculitis in the dog is suggested in one textbook [26] and the authors have strongly suspected this disease in a few cases with eosinophilic pleural effusion.

In human beings, various diseases have been associated with PE [21], and in dogs, some tumors, such as lymphoma and mast cell tumor, have been associated with eosinophilic pulmonary infiltrate [26].

Idiopathic Parenchymal Disorders

Simple PE (Loeffler pneumonia) in human beings is characterized by migratory pulmonary infiltrates accompanied by peripheral eosinophilia [5]. Respiratory symptoms are minimal or absent, and the disease resolves spontaneously within 4 weeks [5]. A parasitic infection or drug reaction is suspected in many cases, but as many as one third of cases do not have a clinically identifiable cause [21]. Although not reported in the veterinary literature, it is the authors' opinion that this condition exists in the dog based on the observation of several cases of acute and transitory canine EBP that are clinically similar to Loeffler pneumonia in human beings.

Human acute eosinophilic pneumonia is thought to be a unique hypersensitivity reaction to an inhaled antigen [5]. The following diagnostic criteria have been suggested: acute febrile illness of less than 5 to 7 days' duration, hypoxemic respiratory failure, diffuse mixed alveolar and interstitial chest radiographic infiltrates, BALF eosinophilia (>25%), no apparent infectious cause, rapid and complete response to corticosteroid therapy, and no relapse after discontinuation of corticosteroid therapy [27]. A correlate of this condition has not yet been described in dogs.

Human idiopathic chronic eosinophilic pneumonia (ICEP) is a rare disorder of unknown cause characterized by chronic cough, respiratory distress, asthenia, alveolar eosinophilia, and characteristic peripheral alveolar infiltrates on imaging [28]. This disorder is highly responsive to oral corticosteroid therapy; however, relapses are frequent when tapering or after stopping therapy [28]. Moreover, some patients develop severe asthma at some time during the course of disease [29]. EBP in dogs shares some clinical features with human ICEP. Eosinophilic inflammation involves the bronchi in most cases of canine EBP, asthenia is usually absent in EBP, and imaging findings in EBP are not as characteristic as in ICEP [4]. Bronchial hyperactivity has been observed in some dogs with EBP, although EBP is not complicated by asthma. Clinically and pathologically, canine EBP resembles a mixture of human EB and ICEP, with some cases predominantly involving the bronchi and others primarily involving the pulmonary parenchyma.

Canine eosinophilic pulmonary granulomatosis is a disease with no real counterpart in human medicine. This clinical condition usually manifests as progressive cough and respiratory distress with anorexia, weight loss, and lethargy [15]. Radiographic abnormalities are characterized by multiple pulmonary masses of various sizes and hilar lymphadenopathy. The granulomas consist of dense accumulations of large epithelioid cells, macrophages, and eosinophils.

Granulomas may also be found in other organs, such as the liver or kidneys [30]. The response to therapy is poor, and most dogs are euthanized shortly after diagnosis [30]. Occult heartworm disease has been implicated in the pathogenesis of disease in some cases; however, a significant proportion of cases are idiopathic [30,31].

ETIOLOGY AND PATHOGENESIS OF CANINE EOSINOPHILIC BRONCHOPNEUMOPATHY

The cause of canine EBP remains unclear, although hypersensitivity to aeroallergens is suspected [4]. In one study, an intradermal skin test using a panel of 48 standardized allergens, including house dust mite; *Dirofilaria pteronyssinus*; *Dirofilaria farinae*; *Tyrophagus*; human dander; mixed feathers; molds; pollens of grasses, trees, and weeds; and mixed insects, was positive in 4 of 12 dogs with untreated EBP [32]. In another study, 3 dogs with EBP were tested with various antigens and all 3 were negative [1]. The relation between positive intradermal skin testing and documentation of aeroallergens responsible for EBP is difficult to establish. A positive intradermal skin test does not necessarily indicate that the allergen identified is responsible for the pulmonary response. This may be explained by such factors as a difference in mast cell distribution between the lungs and skin or in the route of allergen exposure leading to hypersensitivity. Indeed, there is a discrepancy between localized and systemic immune responses after antigen challenge in the lung [33]. Measurement of serum allergen-specific IgE might provide additional insight into the role of aeroallergens in eosinophilic lung disease, but such measurements have not been conducted to date.

Although the etiology of EBP is still unknown, some of the pathogenesis has been elucidated. In canine EBP, a selective increase in CD4+ T cells and a selective decrease in CD8+ T cells have been demonstrated in BALF [32]. In one dog with EBP, an overrepresentation of CD4+ T cells was confirmed by immunohistochemistry in the bronchial mucosa and pulmonary interstitium [34]. This is similar to the situation in human bronchial asthma, EB, and ICEP, wherein the ratio of CD4+ T cells to CD8+ T cells increases and activated T helper (Th) 2 cells accumulate at sites of inflammation [35–39].

Eosinophilic infiltration and a predominance of CD4+ T cells in BALF support the role for a dominant Th2 immune response in the lower airways in dogs with EBP. Despite this, real-time reverse transcriptase (RT) polymerase chain reaction (PCR) has not confirmed a significant difference in bronchial Th2 cytokine expression in dogs with EBP compared with control animals [40]. The lack of a significant difference between control and diseased dogs is thought to be related to the methodology used. First of all, by using mucosal biopsies, mRNA produced in mucosal T cells may have been diluted in the total mRNA produced by mucosal cell types [40]. Second, RT-PCR methods have recently been improved by assessing RNA quantity and quality before doing the PCR and by using multiple internal control genes for calculation of gene expression. These changes have been shown to improve the accuracy of results obtained from canine nasal biopsies [41] and must be used to assess bronchial tissue or BALF from dogs with EBP to provide a definitive conclusion. Another way to evaluate the cytokine profile in lower airways would be to determine the cytokine protein concentrations in BALF by using capture ELISA. Antibodies specific for canine cytokines are currently being developed [42], and this method could be used to characterize the immune response in EBP. Improved understanding of the immunopathogenesis of disease should lead to improved treatment modalities.

Quantification of mRNA encoding for several CC-chemokines and one of their receptors (CCR3) [40] has not revealed a significant difference in expression of monocyte chemoattractant protein (MCP)-1, MCP-2, MCP-4, and CCR3 between control dogs and dogs with EBP. Expression of transcript for MCP-3, eotaxin-2, and eotaxin-3 was significantly greater in bronchial biopsies from dogs with EBP than in samples from control dogs, however, and significantly less mRNA encoding for regulated on activation normal T-cell expressed and secreted protein (RANTES) was found in the mucosa of dogs with EBP [40]. Eotaxins are the strongest chemoattractants for eosinophils and basophils [43]. MCP-3 attracts eosinophils but also other cell types, such as monocytes, dendritic cells, basophils, and T cells [44]. Increased mRNA levels for MCP-3, eotaxin-2, and eotaxin-3 in bronchial biopsies from dogs with EBP suggest that these chemokines drive the recruitment of eosinophils and mononuclear cells into the airways in EBP.

The lower airway and parenchymal destruction and remodeling observed in canine EBP is at least partially related to upregulation of collagenolysis and proteolysis. Indeed, collagenase activity of matrix metalloproteinases (MMPs) is increased in BALF from dogs with EBP as compared with that found in BALF from control animals [2,45]. This increased collagenolytic activity is partially attributable to increased activity of MMP-8, MMP-9, and MMP-13 [2,45]. In EBP, these MMPs seem to be produced by macrophages and epithelial cells and not by eosinophils [2,45]. Epithelial laminins are among the proteins that are degraded by MMPs in canine EBP [46], and increased laminin-5γ2-chain degradation products in BALF from these dogs indicate epithelial injury. Epithelial sloughing leading to temporary denudation of the basement membrane is evident histologically at the bronchial and alveolar levels in canine eosinophilic lung disease [46].

Procollagen type III amino terminal propeptide (PIIINP) is a marker of extracellular matrix turnover [47]. A quantitative test to identify PIIINP has been developed in an attempt to evaluate organ fibrosis. This test is a sensitive but nonspecific marker for assessment of tissue collagen type III turnover [48]. High BALF PIIINP concentrations have been found in dogs with EBP [49]. Although further investigations in large populations of dogs with varying bronchopulmonary pathologic findings are warranted, this study suggests that BALF PIIINP could be a promising marker of lung disease in the dog [49]. Higher PIIINP concentrations in serum and BALF of healthy growing dogs compared with adults might limit the usefulness of PIIINP as a marker of fibrosis in young animals, however.

SIGNALMENT

Dogs affected with EBP are usually young adults (4–6 years of age) [1,2,4,45]. Age at disease onset ranges from 3 months to 13 years, and the interval between disease onset and diagnosis varies from 3 weeks to 6 years [1,2,4]. A breed predisposition for Siberian Huskies and Alaskan Malamutes was present in one study [4], but the disease is found in other large breeds (eg, Labrador Retrievers, Rottweilers, German Shepherds) as well as in small breeds (eg, Fox and Jack Russell Terriers, Dachshunds). The weight of affected dogs varies from 4 to 50 kg [1,2,4]. A gender bias has been reported, with female dogs apparently more frequently affected than male dogs in a proportion of 1.3:3 [2,4,32], although an older study mentions a proportion of 0.5:1 [10]. Interestingly, human patients diagnosed with ICEP are twice as likely to be female [28].

CLINICAL SIGNS

At initial presentation, cough is the most common clinical sign, occurring in 95% to 100% of dogs [1,2,4]. The cough is usually harsh and sonorous, persistent, and frequently followed by gagging and retching. Early in the course of disease, gagging and retching might be confused with a disorder of the digestive tract [4]. Other clinical signs frequently reported include respiratory difficulty and exercise intolerance. Nasal discharge is present in up to 50% of cases; it can be serous, mucoid, or mucopurulent and can be associated with a concomitant eosinophilic rhinitis in some cases [4]. General systemic health is not always affected [1,2,4] unless concomitant disease is present. Pruritus, with or without skin lesions, is another clinical complaint that is occasionally reported [1]. On physical examination, thoracic auscultation can be normal but increased lung sounds, wheezes, or crackles are often found [1,4].

DIAGNOSIS

EBP may be suspected based on signalment, history of a positive response to corticosteroids, and clinical signs. Diagnosis relies on radiographic and bronchoscopic findings, blood eosinophilia, tissue eosinophilic infiltration demonstrated by cytology of BALF or histopathologic examination of bronchial biopsies, and exclusion of known causes of eosinophilic infiltration of the lower airways. The diagnosis of EBP must be confirmed before treatment is initiated, because long-term corticosteroids are needed to control clinical signs of disease in most cases.

Thoracic Radiography

Diffuse radiographic infiltrates of variable intensity are found in dogs with EBP and are generally more severe than those found in dogs with chronic bronchitis. The most frequently encountered pattern is a mixed moderate to severe bronchointerstitial pattern. Peribronchial cuffing is a frequent lesion (in approximately 20% of cases) as well as marked thickening of the bronchial walls [4]. Alveolar infiltration is also common and can be identified in up to 40% of the cases [4,32]. Bronchiectasis is commonly encountered in chronic cases [4,10]. The radiographic severity score correlates significantly with the BALF total cell count and eosinophil count but not with the blood eosinophil count [2]. Radiographic features are illustrated in Fig. 1.

Hematology

Hematologic abnormalities include leukocytosis in 30% to 50% of the cases, eosinophilia in 50% to 60%, neutrophilia in 25% to 30%, and basophilia in 0% to 55% [1,2,4]. Absence of peripheral eosinophilia does not exclude a diagnosis of EBP [4]. Similarly, in people with ICEP, blood eosinophilia is not a constant finding [28]. Dogs with EBP generally have normal serum biochemistry values.

Airway Evaluation

Airway sampling is necessary to confirm a diagnosis of EBP through cytologic assessment and exclusion of infection. Collection of an airway sample by tracheal wash or bronchoscopy can be used to confirm the diagnosis. Bronchoscopy is particularly useful because it allows identification of eosinophilic infiltration in BALF or in mucosal biopsies. Bronchoscopy also allows observation of macroscopic findings typical of EBP and the detection of possible concomitant bacterial infection that requires prompt treatment before initiating therapy for EBP itself. Bronchoscopic examination is performed under general anesthesia, using a flexible bronchoscope.

Bronchoalveolar lavage (BAL) is considered to be a safe procedure in dogs, although in a single case report, a dog with EBP developed severe respiratory distress after BAL, presumably because of eosinophil degranulation and severe bronchoconstriction after BAL. The dog required mechanical ventilation for almost 24 hours along with anti-inflammatory and bronchodilator medications

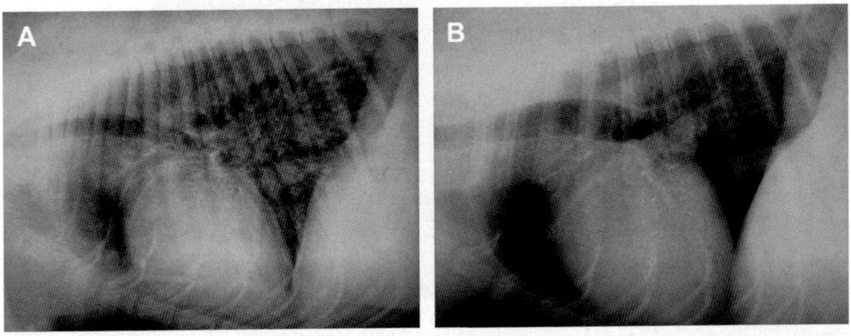

Fig. 1. (A) Right lateral projection of the thorax shows a severe bronchointerstitial pattern in a dog with EBP. (B) The same dog after treatment with oral corticosteroids.

for full recovery [50]. Therefore, careful monitoring of cardiac and respiratory parameters is recommended when performing bronchoscopy, particularly if EBP is suspected.

Macroscopic findings

The macroscopic bronchoscopic features defined in EBP include (1) the presence of a moderate to large amount of yellow-green secretions; (2) mucosal changes, such as moderate to severe thickening of the mucosa with an irregular or polypoid appearance; (3) dramatic airway hyperemia; and (4) less often, exaggerated concentric airway closure during expiration [2,4,32]. Endoscopic features are illustrated in Fig. 2.

Bronchoalveolar lavage

Cytology. BALF must be centrifuged or cytocentrifuged immediately to obtain good-quality cytologic samples. Alternatively, a protected catheter brush can be inserted through the biopsy channel of the bronchoscope to obtain material for cytology. BALF cytology detects local eosinophilic infiltration more reliably

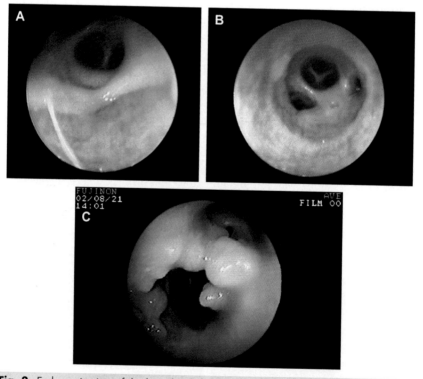

Fig. 2. Endoscopic view of the bronchi of dogs with EBP shows thick yellow material (A), thickening of the mucosa with an irregular surface (B), and polypoid appearance of the mucosa (C).

than brush cytology, and this is likely attributable to the larger area sampled with BAL than with a brush [32]. Using either technique, a cytologic grade can be assigned, based on the percentage of eosinophils. Normal cell counts in BALF range from 200 to 400 cells/µL, with macrophages predominating (65%–70% of the total count). EBP is characterized by an increase in the total number of cells in BALF as well as an increase in the percentage of eosinophils and neutrophils (Fig. 3) [2,4]. Less than 5% eosinophils are generally found in the BALF from healthy dogs, although there seems to be a population of clinically normal dogs with high relative (up to 24%) or absolute eosinophil counts in BALF [2,4,51]. This might be a result of parasitic burden among various facilities or of genetic differences between individuals. Siberian Huskies seem predisposed to a high number of eosinophils in blood and BALF in the absence of obvious clinical signs of inflammation (Cécile Clercx, DVM, PhD, unpublished data, 2000), and care must be taken when interpreting differential cell counts from BALF.

Cytology of BALF can also be helpful to rule out other disease processes; parasitic eggs or larvae, *Toxoplasma gondii* tachyzoites [52], or tumor cells [51] can be detected, and the presence of intracellular bacteria allows identification of an infectious process [53].

Microbiology. The central airways of healthy dogs are not sterile, and in dogs with suspected EBP, it is important to get an accurate assessment of bacteria in the BALF by submitting a quantitative bacterial culture [53]. Pulmonary bacterial infection is uncommon in dogs with EBP, but it should be promptly recognized and treated before initiating therapy with glucocorticoids [32]. It is common for dogs with EBP to have received antibiotic therapy before presentation based on a positive bacterial culture or because of the presence of an

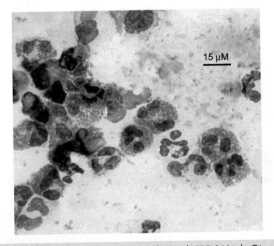

15 µM

Fig. 3. Bronchoalveolar lavage cytology from a dog with EBP (Wright-Giemsa stain, original magnification ×150). The percentage of eosinophils (n = 100) was more than 50%.

alveolar pattern on thoracic radiographs; however, the clinical response is minimal at best.

A fumigatus was cultured from the BALF of two dogs with EBP [4], but because cytology and histopathologic examination failed to identify the organism, these positive cultures were considered contaminants. Fungal culture of BALF is not routinely recommended for dogs with EBP.

Histopathologic findings. Perendoscopic mucosal bronchial biopsies are used for histopathologic examination. Histopathologic findings are graded according to severity: grades 1, 2, and 3 correspond to eosinophilic infiltrate with mild, moderate, and severe inflammatory changes, respectively (Fig. 4) [4]. Hyperplasia, squamous metaplasia, epithelial ulceration, microhemorrhage, hemosiderin-laden macrophages, collagenolysis, and fibrosis can also be seen in grade 3 EBP [4]. Unfortunately, cytologic grade based on BAL analysis and histopathologic grade do not seem to be correlated [4,32].

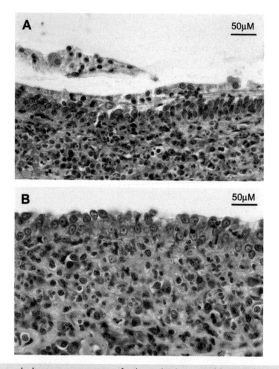

Fig. 4. (A) Histopathologic examination of a bronchial mucosal biopsy from a dog with EBP revealed moderate inflammation (grade 2) with extravasation of eosinophils from superficial mucosal vessels and migration of these cells through the respiratory epithelium into the bronchial lumen (hematoxylin and eosin, original magnification ×187). (B) Eosinophils within the mucosa are accompanied by plasma cells, lymphocytes, macrophages, and mast cells (hematoxylin and eosin, original magnification ×187). (*From* Clercx C, Peeters D, Snaps F, et al. Eosinophilic bronchopneumopathy in dogs. J Vet Intern Med 2000;14(3):282–91; with permission.)

Rhinoscopy

In dogs with concomitant nasal discharge, the nasal cavities should be investigated using a rhinoscope and samples obtained for bacterial and cytologic examinations (brush or imprint cytology). Rhinoscopy may reveal congested and edematous mucosa, mucoid or mucopurulent secretions, and polypoid proliferations in severe cases [4]. Brush cytology or histopathologic examination typically reveals the presence of eosinophils.

Parasitic Analysis

Because eosinophilic pneumonia can be caused by occult heartworm disease [14], it is strongly advised to run a heartworm antigen test in endemic areas or in dogs that have traveled to an endemic area [54].

Helminth parasites are implicated in eosinophilic bronchopulmonary reactions through primary infection or by migration through lung tissue during development [18]. Zinc sulfate centrifugation-flotation and Baermann sedimentation of feces are advised, because these tests detect eggs or larvae for most pulmonary parasites. A negative fecal examination by either method is not conclusive, however, because a single fecal examination detects only 30% to 70% of active infections [55]. It is therefore advised to repeat the fecal examination in suspect cases or to treat against potential parasites using a course of an appropriate antihelminthic (eg, fenbendazole, thiabendazole, levamisole). In these cases, a short course of prednisolone may be required to suppress the associated hypersensitivity reaction.

Intradermal Skin Testing

Searching for potential aeroallergens could be considered as part of a complete investigation of inciting factors for eosinophilic inflammation, although results are open to interpretation. Intradermal skin testing must be performed before treatment with corticosteroids.

Pulmonary Function Tests

Arterial blood gas analysis is a valuable test that provides insights into the severity of pulmonary dysfunction in animals with parenchymal disease. Mild decreased values in PaO_2 and increased values in the alveolar-arterial oxygen gradient (A-aDO_2) have been described in dogs with EBP as compared with healthy animals [2]. Arterial blood gas analysis does not allow differentiation between EBP and other diseases, however.

PFTs are used extensively in human medicine to evaluate and diagnose pulmonary diseases as well as to monitor the response to therapy [56]. This is especially true in allergic or eosinophilic disorders, in which a bronchospastic component is one of the hallmarks of the disease process. Unfortunately, most PFTs require conscious maneuvers (eg, maximal expiration) that are not possible in animals.

Pulmonary mechanics can be investigated by various methods, but most techniques require anesthesia. Static respiratory compliance was measured in five anesthetized dogs with EBP and was decreased in two of them, presumably because of the presence of infiltrates around airways and in the lung parenchyma that made the lung less distensible [1]. Noninvasive PFTs that do not require patient cooperation, and are therefore suitable for clinical purposes; they have been described in dogs in the past few years, including tidal breathing flow volume loops and whole-body barometric plethysmography (BWBP) [57,58]. Tidal breathing flow volume loops have proven useful for detecting upper airway obstruction in conscious dogs [57,59] and have revealed expiratory flow limitation in dogs with bronchitis [57] but have not been examined in dogs with EBP. BWBP is a noninvasive PFT that allows measurement of airway reactivity in unrestrained, conscious, and spontaneously breathing animals [58,60,61]. Based on preliminary assessment of bronchoreactivity using BWBP, it seems that some dogs with EBP may have active bronchoconstriction rather than passive airway collapse (Cécile Clercx, DVM, PhD, unpublished data, 2005). Such measurements need to be performed in a larger number of dogs with EBP before and after treatment to provide definitive conclusions.

TREATMENT

The treatment of choice for canine EBP is oral corticosteroid therapy (methylprednisolone) initiated at a dose of 1 mg/kg administered orally twice daily during the first week. This dose is then given on alternate days during the second week, and further reduced to 1 mg/kg administered orally daily on alternate days during the third week. If clinical signs remain well controlled, the dose is gradually decreased until maintenance levels are achieved [2–4]. In one study, the maintenance dose of prednisolone ranged between 0.125 mg/kg and 0.5 mg/kg every other day or even every 3 or 4 days [4]. The response to steroid therapy is generally good [2–4]. Cough, respiratory difficulty, and exercise intolerance begin to improve within days, although full resolution of clinical signs can take months. Nasal discharge is sometimes more refractory to steroid treatment. During steroid therapy, blood eosinophilia and eosinophilic inflammation in BALF or bronchial biopsies improve or resolve. Radiographic and bronchoscopic scores also improve, although chronic lesions often persist [2,4,32]. Finally, steroid therapy results in normalization of the increased CD4+ T cells/CD8+ T cells found in BALF before treatment [32].

Relapse of clinical signs can occur within weeks or months after drug discontinuation, but some dogs seem to be cured by steroid therapy [1,32]. In a study in which dogs were treated with corticosteroids for 8 weeks, 6 of 20 dogs relapsed and needed immediate reinstitution of therapy [2]. This could indicate that a longer period of tapering medication might be required in some dogs.

The time from onset of clinical signs until diagnosis does not seem to influence the response to treatment, because even patients with chronic or severe forms of EBP showed a positive response to medical therapy. In one report, younger patients were more difficult to manage [26]; however, in the authors' experience, age at the time of diagnosis does not influence the response to treatment [4]. The poorest response to treatment has been reported in cases treated with high doses of glucocorticoids that are abruptly discontinued or in those treated with irregular parenteral administration of depository steroid injections [26].

In most cases, the response to corticosteroid therapy is considered to be satisfactory. Despite a gradual decrease in dosage, however, some animals still require relatively high doses of glucocorticoids to control signs, and weight gain, polyuria or polydipsia, and panting become undesirable side effects. In other animals, the use of glucocorticoids is contraindicated because of health problems, such as diabetes mellitus or obesity. In these cases, inhaled steroids could prove beneficial. Medications given by means of inhalation offer the advantage of high drug concentrations within the airways while attenuating systemic side effects. Inhaled corticosteroids (eg, fluticasone propionate) have been used successfully in cats for the management of experimental bronchitis by utilizing a low-resistance spacer device connected to a face mask [62,63]. A recent study has shown that inhaled corticosteroids can be used for the management of chronic bronchitis and EBP in dogs [64]. Further prospective studies are warranted in larger numbers of animals to define optimum treatment protocols and to investigate potential side effects.

Novel therapies might also need to be considered. Although the role of aeroallergens in EBP is unclear, hyposensitization directed against allergens identified by skin testing has resulted in clinical improvement in rare cases (B.C. McKiernan, unpublished data, 2004). Cyclosporine, a cyclic oligopeptide macrolide that possesses immunomodulating properties, is a drug that has been used successfully in the treatment of canine atopic dermatitis [65]. Although the drug is expensive, it could be an interesting drug to try in dogs with EBP that cannot tolerate glucocorticoids. No trial results are available to date.

Recent advances in molecular biology have enhanced our understanding of the mechanisms by which eosinophils are recruited to the lungs and have led to the discovery of new potential drug targets. New therapeutic strategies based on the use of immunomodulatory substances are being investigated in human patients with bronchial asthma and in murine models of disease. Those medications include (1) drugs that suppress the effects of certain interleukins (ILs), specifically IL-5 [66] or IL-13 [67]; (2) compounds that interfere with the main receptor involved in the recruitment of eosinophils (CCR3) [68,69]; and (3) CpG oligodeoxynucleotides that direct the inflammatory reaction toward a Th1 type [70]. In the future, these novel therapies might be applied to canine EBP.

Several new and intriguing agents that might be useful in eosinophilic lung disease exist on the horizon. Given the remarkable efficacy of oral corticosteroids in the treatment of EBP, however, potential new therapies need to be rigorously proven to be superior to corticosteroids before a change in standard practice is advised [3].

In conclusion, canine EBP is a disease characterized by eosinophilic infiltration of the lung and bronchial mucosa. Although the etiology of EBP is still unknown, the presence of eosinophilic infiltration and a predominance of CD4+ T cells suggest a Th2 immune response mounted in the lower airways.

Hypersensitivity to aeroallergens must be considered as a potential etiology. Additional studies of the tissue cytokine expression profile and of allergen-specific IgE are needed to confirm this hypothesis. The prognosis for dogs with EBP is usually good, because the response to oral corticosteroid therapy is excellent in most cases, although systemic side effects of steroids can be limiting.

References

[1] Corcoran BM, Thoday KL, Henfrey JI, et al. Pulmonary infiltration with eosinophils in 14 Dogs. J Small Anim Pract 1991;32(10):494–502.

[2] Rajamaki MM, Jarvinen AK, Sorsa T, et al. Clinical findings, bronchoalveolar lavage fluid cytology and matrix metalloproteinase-2 and -9 in canine pulmonary eosinophilia. Vet J 2002;163(2):168–81.

[3] Norris C, Mellema M. Eosinophilic pneumonia. In: King L, editor. Textbook of respiratory disease in dogs and cats. St Louis (MO): Saunders; 2004. p. 541–7.

[4] Clercx C, Peeters D, Snaps F, et al. Eosinophilic bronchopneumopathy in dogs. J Vet Intern Med 2000;14(3):282–91.

[5] Alberts WM. Eosinophilic interstitial lung disease. Curr Opin Pulm Med 2004;10(5): 419–24.

[6] Shepherd JM, Duddleston DN, Hicks GS, et al. Asthma: a brief overview. Am J Med Sci 2002;324(4):174–9.

[7] Brightling CE, Symon FA, Birring SS, et al. Comparison of airway immunopathology of eosinophilic bronchitis and asthma. Thorax 2003;58(6):528–32.

[8] Dicpinigaitis PV. Cough. 4: cough in asthma and eosinophilic bronchitis. Thorax 2004; 59(1):71–2.

[9] Park SW, Lee YM, Jang AS, et al. Development of chronic airway obstruction in patients with eosinophilic bronchitis: a prospective follow-up study. Chest 2004;125(6): 1998–2004.

[10] Brownlie SE. A retrospective study of diagnoses in 109 cases of canine lower respiratory-disease. J Small Anim Pract 1990;31(8):371–6.

[11] Zander DS. Allergic bronchopulmonary aspergillosis: an overview. Arch Pathol Lab Med 2005;129(7):924–8.

[12] Katzenstein AL, Liebow AA, Friedman PJ. Bronchocentric granulomatosis, mucoid impaction, and hypersensitivity reactions to fungi. Am Rev Respir Dis 1975;111(4):497–537.

[13] van der Klooster JM, Nurmohamed LA, van Kaam NA. Bronchocentric granulomatosis associated with influenza-A virus infection. Respiration 2004;71(4):412–6.

[14] Calvert CA, Losonsky JM. Pneumonitis associated with occult heartworm disease in dogs. J Am Vet Med Assoc 1985;186(10):1097–8.

[15] Calvert CA. Eosinophilic pulmonary granulomatosis. In: Kirk R, Bonagura J, editors. Current veterinary therapy XI. Philadelphia: WB Saunders; 1992. p. 813–6.

[16] Martin MWS, Ashton G, Simpson VR, et al. Angiostrongylosis in Cornwall—clinical presentations of 8 cases. J Small Anim Pract 1993;34(1):20–5.

[17] Chapman P, Boag A, Guitian J, et al. Angiostrongylus vasorum infection in 23 dogs (1999–2002). J Small Anim Pract 2004;45:435–40.

[18] Taboada J. Pulmonary diseases of potential allergic origin. Semin Vet Med Surg (Small Anim) 1991;6(4):278–85.

[19] Noone K. Pulmonary hypersensitivities. In: Kirk R, editor. Current veterinary therapy IX. Philadelphia: WB Saunders; 1986. p. 285–92.

[20] Corcoran BM, Cobb M, Martin MW, et al. Chronic pulmonary disease in West Highland white terriers. Vet Rec 1999;144(22):611–6.

[21] Allen JN, Davis WB. Eosinophilic lung diseases. Am J Respir Crit Care Med 1994;150(5 Pt 1): 1423–38.

[22] Weller PF, Bubley GJ. The idiopathic hypereosinophilic syndrome. Blood 1994;83(10): 2759–79.

[23] Aroch I, Perl S, Markovics A. Disseminated eosinophilic disease resembling idiopathic hypereosinophilic syndrome in a dog. Vet Rec 2001;149(13):386–9.

[24] Sykes JE, Weiss DJ, Buoen LC, et al. Idiopathic hypereosinophilic syndrome in 3 Rottweilers. J Vet Intern Med 2001;15(2):162–6.

[25] Perkins M, Watson A. Successful treatment of hypereosinophilic syndrome in a dog. Aust Vet J 2001;79(10):686–9.

[26] Bauer T. Pulmonary hypersensitivity disorders. In: Kirk R, editor. Current veterinary therapy X. Philadelphia: WB Saunders; 1989. p. 369–76.

[27] Pope-Harman AL, Davis WB, Allen ED, et al. Acute eosinophilic pneumonia. A summary of 15 cases and review of the literature. Medicine (Baltimore) 1996;75(6):334–42.

[28] Marchand E, Reynaud-Gaubert M, Lauque D, et al. Idiopathic chronic eosinophilic pneumonia. A clinical and follow-up study of 62 cases. The Groupe d'Etudes et de Recherche sur les Maladies "Orphelines" Pulmonaires (GERM"O""P"). Medicine (Baltimore) 1998;77(5): 299–312.

[29] Marchand E, Etienne-Mastroianni B, Chanez P, et al. Idiopathic chronic eosinophilic pneumonia and asthma: how do they influence each other? Eur Respir J 2003;22(1): 8–13.

[30] Calvert CA, Mahaffey MB, Lappin MR, et al. Pulmonary and disseminated eosinophilic granulomatosis in dogs. J Am Anim Hosp Assoc 1988;24(3):311–20.

[31] von Rotz A, Suter MM, Mettler F, et al. Eosinophilic granulomatous pneumonia in a dog. Vet Rec 1986;118(23):631–2.

[32] Clercx C, Peeters D, German AJ, et al. An immunologic investigation of canine eosinophilic bronchopneumopathy. J Vet Intern Med 2002;16(3):229–37.

[33] Bice DE, Jones SE, Muggenburg BA. Long-term antibody production after lung immunization and challenge: role of lung and lymphoid tissues. Am J Respir Cell Mol Biol 1993;8(6): 662–7.

[34] Peeters D, Day MJ, Clercx C. An immunohistochemical study of canine eosinophilic bronchopneumopathy. J Comp Pathol 2005;133(2–3):128–35.

[35] Brightling CE, Symon FA, Birring SS, et al. T(H)2 cytokine expression in bronchoalveolar lavage fluid T lymphocytes and bronchial submucosa is a feature of asthma and eosinophilic bronchitis. J Allergy Clin Immunol 2002;110(6):899–905.

[36] Robinson DS, Bentley AM, Hartnell A, et al. Activated memory T helper cells in bronchoalveolar lavage fluid from patients with atopic asthma: relation to asthma symptoms, lung function, and bronchial responsiveness. Thorax 1993;48(1):26–32.

[37] Robinson DS, Hamid Q, Ying S, et al. Predominant Th2-like bronchoalveolar T-lymphocyte population in atopic asthma. N Engl J Med 1992;326(5):298–304.

[38] Walker C, Bauer W, Braun RK, et al. Activated T cells and cytokines in bronchoalveolar lavages from patients with various lung diseases associated with eosinophilia. Am J Respir Crit Care Med 1994;150(4):1038–48.

[39] Albera C, Ghio P, Solidoro P, et al. Activated and memory alveolar T-lymphocytes in idiopathic eosinophilic pneumonia. Eur Respir J 1995;8(8):1281–5.

[40] Peeters D, Peters IR, Clercx C, et al. Real-time RT-PCR quantification of mRNA encoding cytokines, CC chemokines and CCR3 in bronchial biopsies from dogs with eosinophilic bronchopneumopathy. Vet Immunol Immunopathol 2006;110(1-2):65–77.

[41] Peeters D, Peters IR, Helps CR, et al. Distinct tissue cytokine and chemokine mRNA expression in canine sino-nasal aspergillosis and idiopathic lymphoplasmacytic rhinitis. Vet Immunol Immunopathol 2007;117(1-2):95–105. doi:10.1016/vetimm.2007.01.018.

[42] de Lima VM, Peiro JR, de Oliveira Vasconcelos R. IL-6 and TNF-alpha production during active canine visceral leishmaniasis. Vet Immunol Immunopathol 2007;115(1–2): 189–93.

[43] Lloyd C. Chemokines in allergic lung inflammation. Immunology 2002;105(2):144–54.

[44] Lukacs NW. Role of chemokines in the pathogenesis of asthma. Nat Rev Immunol 2001;1(2):108–16.

[45] Rajamaki MM, Jarvinen AK, Sorsa T, et al. Collagenolytic activity in bronchoalveolar lavage fluid in canine pulmonary eosinophilia. J Vet Intern Med 2002;16(6):658–64.

[46] Rajamaki MM, Jarvinen AK, Sorsa TA, et al. Elevated levels of fragmented laminin-5 gamma2-chain in bronchoalveolar lavage fluid from dogs with pulmonary eosinophilia. Vet J 2006;171(3):562–5.

[47] Risteli L, Risteli J. Analysis of extracellular matrix proteins in biological fluids. Methods Enzymol 1987;145:391–411.

[48] Jensen LT. The aminoterminal propeptide of type III procollagen. Studies on physiology and pathophysiology. Dan Med Bull 1997;44(1):70–8.

[49] Schuller S, Valentin S, Remy B, et al. Analytical, physiologic, and clinical validation of a radioimmunoassay for measurement of procollagen type III amino terminal propeptide in serum and bronchoalveolar lavage fluid obtained from dogs. Am J Vet Res 2006;67(5): 749–55.

[50] Cooper ES, Schober KE, Drost WT. Severe bronchoconstriction after bronchoalveolar lavage in a dog with eosinophilic airway disease. J Am Vet Med Assoc 2005;227(8): 1257–62.

[51] Hawkins EC, DeNicola DB, Kuehn NF. Bronchoalveolar lavage in the evaluation of pulmonary disease in the dog and cat. State of the art. J Vet Intern Med 1990;4(5):267–74.

[52] Hawkins EC, Davidson MG, Meuten DJ, et al. Cytologic identification of toxoplasma gondii in bronchoalveolar lavage fluid of experimentally infected cats. J Am Vet Med Assoc 1997;210(5):648–50.

[53] Peeters DE, McKiernan BC, Weisiger RM, et al. Quantitative bacterial cultures and cytological examination of bronchoalveolar lavage specimens in dogs. J Vet Intern Med 2000;14(5):534–41.

[54] Atkins C. Canine heartworm disease. In: Ettinger S, Feldman E, editors. Textbook of veterinary internal medicine. St. Louis (MO): Elsevier Saunders; 2005. p. 1118–36.

[55] Sherding R. Parasites of the lung. In: King L, editor. Textbook of respiratory diseases in dogs and cats. St. Louis (MO): Saunders; 2004. p. 548–59.

[56] Crapo RO. Pulmonary-function testing. N Engl J Med 1994;331(1):25–30.

[57] Amis TC, Kurpershoek C. Tidal breathing flow-volume loop analysis for clinical assessment of airway obstruction in conscious dogs. Am J Vet Res 1986;47(5):1002–6.

[58] Talavera J, Kirschvink N, Schuller S, et al. Evaluation of respiratory function by barometric whole-body plethysmography in healthy dogs. Vet J 2006;172(1):67–77.

[59] Amis TC, Smith MM, Gaber CE, et al. Upper airway obstruction in canine laryngeal paralysis. Am J Vet Res 1986;47(5):1007–10.

[60] Hoffman AM, Dhupa N, Cimetti L. Airway reactivity measured by barometric whole-body plethysmography in healthy cats. Am J Vet Res 1999;60(12):1487–92.

[61] Kirschvink N, Leemans J, Delvaux F, et al. Non-invasive assessment of growth, gender and time of day related changes of respiratory pattern in healthy cats by use of barometric whole body plethysmography. Vet J 2006;172(3):446–54.

[62] Reinero CR, Decile KC, Byerly JR, et al. Effects of drug treatment on inflammation and hyperreactivity of airways and on immune variables in cats with experimentally induced asthma. Am J Vet Res 2005;66(7):1121–7.

[63] Kirschvink N, Leemans J, Delvaux F, et al. Inhaled fluticasone reduces bronchial responsiveness and airway inflammation in cats with mild chronic bronchitis. J Feline Med Surg 2006;8(1):45–54.

[64] Bexfield NH, Foale RD, Davison LJ, et al. Management of 13 cases of canine respiratory disease using inhaled corticosteroids. J Small Anim Pract 2006;47(7):377–82.

[65] Steffan J, Favrot C, Mueller R. A systematic review and meta-analysis of the efficacy and safety of cyclosporin for the treatment of atopic dermatitis in dogs. Vet Dermatol 2006; 17(1):3–16.

[66] Kips JC, Tournoy KG, Pauwels RA. New anti-asthma therapies: suppression of the effect of interleukin (IL)-4 and IL-5. Eur Respir J 2001;17(3):499–506.
[67] Zimmermann N, Hershey GK, Foster PS, et al. Chemokines in asthma: cooperative interaction between chemokines and IL-13. J Allergy Clin Immunol 2003;111(2):227–42.
[68] Shen HH, Xu F, Zhang GS, et al. CCR3 monoclonal antibody inhibits airway eosinophilic inflammation and mucus overproduction in a mouse model of asthma. Acta Pharmacol Sin 2006;27(12):1594–9.
[69] Fortin M, Ferrari N, Higgins ME, et al. Effects of antisense oligodeoxynucleotides targeting CCR3 on the airway response to antigen in rats. Oligonucleotides 2006;16(3):203–12.
[70] Hessel EM, Chu M, Lizcano JO, et al. Immunostimulatory oligonucleotides block allergic airway inflammation by inhibiting Th2 cell activation and IgE-mediated cytokine induction. J Exp Med 2005;202(11):1563–73.

Interstitial Lung Diseases

Carol R. Reinero, DVM, PhD*, Leah A. Cohn, DVM, PhD

Department of Veterinary Medicine and Surgery, University of Missouri-Columbia College of
Veterinary Medicine, 379 East Campus Drive, Clydesdale Hall, Columbia, MO 65211, USA

D isorders of the pulmonary parenchyma are frequently diagnosed in dogs and cats. Infectious pneumonia (bacterial, fungal, viral, protozoal, parasitic, or rickettsial in origin) and neoplasia (primary or metastatic) are common causes of parenchymal disease. Interstitial lung diseases (ILDs) are a heterogeneous group of noninfectious nonmalignant respiratory tract disorders that have overlapping clinicopathologic and radiographic features. These are classified as restrictive lung diseases, because inflammation, fibrosis, or abnormal accumulations of protein or lipid reduce effective lung volume and diminish pulmonary compliance. Compared with infectious pneumonia and neoplasia, these diseases are rare, require histopathologic examination for definitive diagnosis, and are generally poorly characterized in small animal patients. Although recognition of ILDs is increasing, they remain underdiagnosed in dogs and cats. The optimal treatment regimen and an accurate prognosis are unknown for many ILDs, and morbidity and mortality may be high.

IMMUNOPATHOGENESIS

The ILDs are associated with disruption of the distal pulmonary parenchyma, with disease involving the interstitium (ie, anatomic space between the basement membrane of the alveolar epithelial cells and capillary endothelial cells) as well as local perivascular and lymphatic tissues. Many of the ILDs arise from injury to the alveolar epithelial lining, which triggers a host inflammatory response and reparative events that lead to structural changes, often including fibrosis. The injury can be secondary to inhalation of pulmonary toxicants, allergens, mineral fibers, or dusts, or it may be caused by vascular damage from drugs, toxins, or immune disease. The cause of ILDs in human beings is frequently unknown, in which no specific cause of the injury is ever identified (ie, idiopathic). This is likely true in dogs and cats as well.

The pulmonary inflammatory cascade triggered by parenchymal injury is intended to repair and restore normal function to the tissue. Chronic inflammation and fibrosis associated with ILDs are a result of dysregulated and exaggerated host tissue repair; however, the self-limiting inflammatory response has been

*Corresponding author. E-mail address: reineroc@missouri.edu (C.R. Reinero).

0195-5616/07/$ – see front matter
doi:10.1016/j.cvsm.2007.05.008

replaced by a cycle of inflammation and collagen deposition. Cells of the innate and adaptive immune system work in concert to orchestrate the chronic changes seen in ILDs. Initially, when tissue is injured, elaboration of vasoactive and chemotactic molecules enables leukocyte infiltration into the damaged pulmonary parenchyma. Neutrophils are the earliest inflammatory cell to arrive at the site of injury. These cells rely on cell adhesion molecules to localize in the pulmonary vasculature and on chemoattractants to gain access to the interstitium and alveolar spaces. Neutrophils contain a variety of preformed toxic particles in their granules (eg, elastase, cathepsin G, collagenase) and can generate toxic oxygen radicals that cause further tissue damage and attract other inflammatory cells. In some ILDs, eosinophils are important mediators of tissue damage and are also attracted to sites of injury or inflammation by chemoattractants. Degranulation of eosinophils causes release of a wide variety of inflammatory mediators, and these cells are postulated to be of critical importance in type I hypersensitivity diseases (eg, eosinophilic pneumonias) in the lung. Macrophages are also attracted to sites of tissue injury and can elaborate a wide range of proinflammatory and profibrotic cytokines. They play a key role in regulation of the fibrotic response, allowing for a net accumulation of collagen (ie, an increase in collagen synthesis and a decrease in collagen degradation) in diseases like idiopathic pulmonary fibrosis (IPF). Lymphocytes are also recognized in cytologic or histologic specimens from patients with some ILDs. T lymphocytes, in particular, may be critical in the modulation of inflammation and fibrosis by virtue of the cytokines they secrete. They are also central players in type IV hypersensitivity (delayed type hypersensitivity [DTH]) pneumonitis.

INTERSTITIAL LUNG DISEASES RECOGNIZED IN DOGS AND CATS

Although there are more than 200 different specific causes of ILDs in human beings, only a limited number of ILDs have been described in dogs and cats. Most of these have been reported in the literature as single case reports and include eosinophilic pneumonia, pulmonary interstitial fibrosis (including IPF), lymphocytic interstitial pneumonitis (LIP), bronchiolitis obliterans with organizing pneumonia (BOOP), endogenous lipid pneumonia (EnLP), pulmonary alveolar proteinosis (PAP), silicosis, and asbestosis [1–10]. More recently, larger case series of some ILDs have been published in dogs and cats. Although these series have been useful in characterizing these diseases in small animals [11–16], only some of the larger studies based inclusion criteria on histologic features. Histologic characterization is the "gold standard" for diagnosis of ILDs in people [12,14–16]. More recently, high-resolution CT (HRCT) has become a critical and routine component of the diagnostic workup of ILDs in human patients. Because histologic features have been correlated with HRCT (concurrent with other clinicopathologic) features, lung biopsy is no longer required in many cases in human medicine [17]. In small animal patients, we are still a long way away from being able to use this multidisciplinary approach to avoid lung biopsy; until there are clear clinical, imaging, and histologic criteria to diagnose and stage ILDs, pathologic examination is fundamental in enhancing the understanding of ILDs in dogs and cats.

Eosinophilic pneumonia has been called pulmonary infiltrates with eosinophilia or eosinophils, eosinophilic bronchopneumopathy, pulmonary hypersensitivity, eosinophilic granulomatous pneumonia, pulmonary eosinophilic granulomatosis, hypereosinophilic syndrome (HES), and eosinophilic pneumonitis in the veterinary literature [1,11,18–22]. It is characterized by a predominant eosinophilic infiltrate of the terminal bronchioles, alveoli, and blood vessels. As indicated by the variety of names applied to this syndrome, there is poor agreement about how the disease should be classified in dogs and cats. In people, the etiology of eosinophilic pneumonia is broadly categorized as being of undetermined origin or of determined origin. Eosinophilic pneumonia of undetermined origin is subdivided into cases of systemic disease with pulmonary involvement (eg, HES) and cases with pulmonary involvement only (eg, chronic eosinophilic pneumonia [CEP]). Eosinophilic pneumonia of determined origin has been subdivided into pneumonia caused by parasitic infection, fungal infection, or other infectious agents and drug-induced pneumonia. This classification system has been reviewed by Peeters and Clercx elsewhere [1] as well as in chapter 6 of this issue.

The term *idiopathic pulmonary fibrosis* is defined by histologic criteria—specifically, a morphologic pattern of usual interstitial pneumonia (UIP). The histologic features of UIP include interstitial fibrosis, fibroblast and myofibroblast proliferation, enlarged air spaces lined by prominent epithelium (so-called "honeycombing"), and relatively mild inflammatory changes [23]. Additionally, there is heterogeneity in the location of remodeling changes and in the time course of lesion development throughout the lungs. IPF has been described in cats and dogs [12–14,23–25]. There is compelling evidence that the disease identified in cats is clinically and pathologically similar to a familial form of the disease in human beings, in which there is a defect in the type II pneumocyte [12,23]. The disease identified in a group of West Highland White Terriers is speculated to be a result of aberrant collagen regulation, and there are differences in the pathologic findings in this breed from what is seen in human beings (ie, these dogs lack fibroblastic foci and honeycombing) [26]. The cause of IPF is unknown, but current theories suggest that IPF results from multiple episodes of epithelial cell activation from unidentified endogenous or exogenous stimuli [27]. Epithelial cell activation, in turn, allows for migration, proliferation, and activation of mesenchymal cells, leading to fibroblastic and myofibroblastic foci.

LIP became more frequently diagnosed in people with the advent of HIV infection. Cats with feline immunodeficiency virus (FIV) have also been described to develop a lymphocytic alveolitis with features of LIP [3]. It is speculated that lentiviruses infect alveolar macrophages and that alveolar T cells are activated, contributing to the pathologic findings in ILD. Despite the fact that LIP has been recognized in cats with FIV infection, it does not seem to be a significant contributor to morbidity or mortality.

BOOP results from injury to distal airways (bronchioles) that become plugged with connective tissue, leading to a downstream organizing pneumonia. In human beings, BOOP is usually idiopathic but can occur secondary to infections, drug reactions, organ transplantation, or inhalation of toxic fumes. Naturally developing BOOP has been described in dogs and a cat [4,14], and experimentally induced BOOP (induced by administration of oleic acid or by infection with adenovirus or *Mycoplasma*) has been described in dogs [16,28,29]. In one naturally developing case, the dog and owner shared the same environment and developed similar clinical manifestations of disease, prompting speculation that the ILD resulted from environmental toxin inhalation [4].

EnLP described in dogs and cats is characterized by interstitial fibrosis and accumulation of giant cells, intra-alveolar fibroplasia, and type II pneumocyte proliferation [8,15,30]. Lesions develop when pneumocytes are injured (generally from inflammatory or neoplastic obstructive lung disease) and undergo degeneration, leading to release of cholesterol and proliferation of type II pneumocytes that overproduce surfactant with a high cholesterol content. Phagocytosis of lipids by alveolar macrophages results in the classic "lipid-laden macrophages" that fill alveolar spaces.

PAP is considered an ILD despite minimal interstitial inflammation and fibrosis and overall general preservation of lung architecture [31]. In this disease, alveoli are diffusely filled with abnormal surfactant components, phospholipids, and cellular debris, leading to diffusion impairment and ventilation-perfusion mismatch. In human beings, the defect is believed to be related to abnormalities in the granulocyte-macrophage colony-stimulating factor (GM-CSF) pathway that normally stimulates differentiation of macrophages. Lack of the receptor-mediated response results in dysfunction of alveolar macrophages and impaired surfactant clearance. In the veterinary literature, PAP has been reported in two dogs, but the role of cytokines was not investigated in either case [9,10].

Silicosis and asbestosis develop after exposure to inhaled organic dusts. Granulomatous interstitial pneumonia with fibrosis follows chronic exposure [5,6]. Silicosis has more commonly been reported in horses in geographic regions in which the soil is rich in silicates (ie, the Monterey-Carmel Peninsula in California) [32] but has also been reported in two dogs, with one living in an industrial/mining region [5]. Asbestosis was reported in a terrier dog kept for killing rats in an asbestos factory in the 1930s [6]. Special studies, such as electron microscopy and x-ray diffraction analysis, are required to characterize the type of crystalline particles observed on histopathologic examination.

DIAGNOSIS OF INTERSTITIAL LUNG DISEASES
Signalment
Most dogs and cats with ILDs are middle aged to older (with the exception of eosinophilic pneumonia, which often occurs in younger animals), and both genders are affected. The ILDs encompass a large number of different syndromes, but some breed predispositions have been recognized. For example, pulmonary

fibrosis has been documented with high frequency in West Highland White Terriers and Staffordshire Bull Terriers [2,13], and eosinophilic pneumonia is reportedly common in Siberian Huskies and has also been recognized in conjunction with HES in Rottweilers [11,22]. Perhaps because reports of ILDs in small animals are sparse, other breed predispositions have not yet been recognized.

History

A thorough history should provide information about clinical signs and the duration of disease (ie, if clinical signs are acute, subacute, or chronic). Most recognized ILDs in dogs have a subacute to chronic course; however, an acute course has been described in dogs with eosinophilic pneumonia [19,20]. Cats are notoriously adept at hiding signs of respiratory disease until significant pulmonary compromise is present; for this reason, the clinical course of chronic ILDs, such as the reported IPF-like syndrome, may seem to be acute [12]. Knowing if the clinical signs are static or progressive may also be helpful in determining differential diagnoses; most ILDs have a progressive course. A history of systemic clinical signs (eg, weight loss, lethargy) indicates that the diagnostic workup should include tests of body systems outside the respiratory tract.

Owners should be questioned about travel history. For example, regionally distributed fungal infections may result in pneumonia with an eosinophilic component [1]. Owners should also be asked about their pets' exposure to potential pulmonary toxicants or irritants, such as inhaled chemical fumes, mineral fibers, dusts, or allergens. Aspiration of mineral oil or petroleum-based products and exposure to bleomycin or the herbicide paraquat might also lead to an ILD.

Clinical and Physical Examination Signs

Clinical signs relating to the respiratory tract in dogs and cats with ILDs include cough, tachypnea or excessive panting, respiratory distress, exercise intolerance, syncope, cyanosis, and hemoptysis [2,12–15]. Respiratory clinical signs may also be absent, especially in cats [12,15]. Nonrespiratory signs, including fever, lethargy, anorexia, and weight loss, are sometimes present [12,14,15]. On physical examination, a spontaneous or elicited cough that is productive or nonproductive may be noted. Adventitial lung sounds may be auscultated; the presence of harsh lung sounds in the absence of an alveolar radiographic pattern is characteristic of IPF in dogs. The absence of adventitial lung sounds does not exclude an ILD. Increased respiratory rate or effort and occasional cyanosis may be observed.

Diagnostic Testing

Hematologic, biochemical, serologic, and fecal tests are frequently performed as initial noninvasive screening tests in animals with respiratory disease. The complete blood cell count may provide evidence for underlying infection (eg, monocytosis with fungal infection, eosinophilia with parasitic infection).

Importantly, peripheral eosinophilia does not always accompany eosinophilic pneumonia. There are no specific findings on the serum biochemical profile suggestive of any ILD. Hyperglobulinemia associated with chronic antigenic stimulation is sometimes recognized. Serology can be important to help diagnose specific fungal, rickettsial, protozoal, viral, and parasitic infectious processes that can mimic ILDs. Serology may also identify an infectious agent predisposing to development of an ILD, for example, FIV, which is associated with LIP in cats, and heartworm or fungal infection, which may lead to eosinophilic pneumonia [1,3]. Similarly, fecal testing may identify various parasitic infections that mimic or contribute to the development of an ILD.

Thoracic radiography is an excellent screening test to identify abnormalities within the lung and to characterize infiltrates according to pattern and distribution. As suggested by its name, most ILDs demonstrate an interstitial pattern, although alveolar patterns are also common (especially when disease is severe) and bronchointerstitial patterns also occur. Nodules may be evident, and hilar lymphadenopathy can be a feature in some ILDs. Because ILDs are restrictive lung diseases, hypoinflation of the lungs is often appreciated. Despite the myriad of changes that may be present, it is important to realize that thoracic radiographs cannot be used to diagnose an ILD definitively. In human medicine, HRCT can provide specific information on the extent, pattern, and location of disease, and specific findings have shown excellent correlation with histopathologic lesions in several ILDs. In fact, HRCT findings, along with clinical evaluation, have negated the need for lung biopsy for diagnosis of many ILDs in human patients [17]. In veterinary medicine, HRCT has been used to identify pulmonary lesions in a series of dogs with presumptive IPF and in a dog with BOOP [4,33]; however, only the dog with BOOP had histopathologic evaluation for confirmation of disease. Further information is required to determine the utility of CT in the diagnosis of ILDs in dogs and cats.

Although not specifically useful in confirmation of ILDs, other diagnostic tests may be indicated. Dogs with IPF tend to be older terriers with cough, exercise intolerance, and crackles on thoracic auscultation. A heart murmur and signs of right-sided heart failure can be detected when severe disease leads to cor pulmonale. Valvular endocardiosis is an important differential diagnosis, and echocardiography can be used to assess cardiac structure and function. Additionally, Doppler echocardiography can be used to assess pulmonary arterial pressures when tricuspid regurgitation or pulmonic insufficiency is present and can objectively document pulmonary hypertension found in association with restrictive lung disease. Arterial blood gas analysis can objectively quantify hypoxemia and the degree of pulmonary dysfunction. Ultimately, invasive diagnostic tests are required to discriminate ILDs from other lung diseases.

Cytologic and microbiologic assessment of pulmonary specimens is most useful to identify infectious and neoplastic causes of lung disease. Although pulmonary fine-needle aspiration (FNA) is usually safe and can be useful in the diagnosis of various types of lung disease [34], it plays only a limited role in the diagnosis of ILDs. Cytologic assessment of samples obtained by FNA can sometimes identify neoplastic cells or infectious microbes; however, absence of these cells does not completely rule out either condition. For most dogs and cats with noninfectious nonneoplastic ILDs, cytologic preparations from FNA are poorly cellular or demonstrate nonspecific inflammatory cells. Blinded or bronchoscopically guided bronchoalveolar lavage can be used to collect specimens for cytology and culture of deep pulmonary tissues. As with FNA, cytologic examination of lavage fluid has its limitations, including an inability to characterize architectural changes in the lung that characterize many ILDs.

Ultimately, lung biopsy is the only definitive means for diagnosis of most noninfectious nonneoplastic ILDs in dogs and cats. The value of lung biopsy in the diagnosis of respiratory tract disease in dogs and cats with nondiagnostic thoracic radiography and bronchoalveolar lavage fluid cytology has been previously described [35,36]. Only biopsy can demonstrate features (eg, fibrosis) characteristic of many ILDs. Lung biopsy may be obtained by a keyhole surgical technique, by thoracoscopy, or by full thoracotomy. The procurement and utility of transbronchial biopsies obtained by means of fiberoptic bronchoscopy are not well described in dogs and cats, although they are frequently used in human patients with ILDs. Lung biopsy in animals with ILDs is essential to confirm the diagnosis, select appropriate therapy, and guide the clinician in giving an appropriate prognosis to owners.

TREATMENT OF INTERSTITIAL LUNG DISEASES

Because ILDs represent a diverse group of diseases, there is no single treatment. If an inciting cause can be identified (eg, fungal infection, parasitic infection), it should be addressed directly when possible. Additional therapy is often aimed at the cycle of inflammation and fibrosis. Supportive therapy with supplemental oxygen support is required for patients with such severe disease that oxygenation is compromised. Specific therapy varies depending on the particular ILD, and for many ILDs in dogs and cats, the optimal therapy has not yet been established.

Treatment of any underlying infectious agent is critical to the treatment of eosinophilic pneumonias. Infection with *Dirofilaria immitis* should be treated with the appropriate adulticide and microfilaricide, and anthelminthics can be administered to dogs and cats with such parasites as *Strongyloides* spp, *Toxocara* spp, and *Ancylostoma* spp. Although not a common sequela to chronic bacterial or fungal infections, eosinophilic pneumonia can develop as a hypersensitivity to these organisms, and appropriate antibiotic and antifungal therapy should be given when diagnosed. If eosinophilic pneumonia develops after introduction of a novel drug, that drug should be discontinued in case it is inducing pulmonary hypersensitivity. When neoplasia (most commonly, lymphoma and mast cell tumor) is implicated in pulmonary eosinophilia, appropriate treatment of the neoplasm should ameliorate signs of pneumonia. If the underlying trigger of pulmonary hypersensitivity is found and addressed, no further therapy may be required. If pulmonary eosinophilia fails to resolve or no underlying cause is identified, immunosuppression is indicated. Prednisone at a dose of 1 to 2mg/kg/d has been previously advocated [11,21]. Other immunosuppressive agents, including cyclophosphamide and azathioprine, have been used in severely affected dogs [18]. For most cases of eosinophilic pneumonia, with appropriate therapy, the prognosis is fair to excellent.

Treatment of pulmonary fibrosis, more specifically, canine IPF and feline IPF-like syndrome, has been frustrating. Glucocorticoids and cytotoxic agents have most commonly been used to treat this condition in dogs and cats; however, as in human patients, there is no clear evidence that any of these therapies improves survival or quality of life. When cough is severe, pharmacologic suppression may improve the quality of life for the dog and owner. Because of the severity of pulmonary hypertension, this complication may need to be addressed directly. The prognosis for animals with ILD depends, in part, on the stage of disease and on how rapidly it is progressing, but the long-term outcome is poor. Most dogs succumb within 18 months of initial clinical signs, and many cats die within weeks of diagnosis [2,12,13,25].

Published reports characterizing LIP, EnLP, silicosis, and asbestosis were derived from necropsy specimens, and as such, no information about the antemortem treatment of these disorders in small animals is available [3,5,6,8,15]. It seems obvious that underlying triggers (eg, FIV infection in cats) or inhalation of silicates and asbestosis should be avoided. Additionally, because obstructive pulmonary disease predisposes to EnLP, direct treatment of infectious, noninfectious inflammatory, neoplastic, and thromboembolic disease is warranted. For cases of LIP and EnLP in cats, the reported lung lesions did not seem to be a significant contributor to death but, more likely, should be considered indicators of other severe underlying or concurrent disease [3,15]. For the reported cases of silicosis, lesions may have contributed to death [5], and for the case of asbestosis, lesions were end stage [6]. The prognosis for these ILDs is unclear in general, and further studies in larger numbers of animals need to be performed.

BOOP has been reported in pet dogs (n = 3) and in a cat [4,14]. It has also been induced experimentally in research dogs administered oleic acid or infected with adenovirus or *Mycoplasma* [16,28,29]. No treatment information was available for the research dogs. The recommended therapy for BOOP in dogs is prednisone at immunosuppressive doses (Fig. 1). One dog with naturally developing BOOP was considered cured after receiving immunosuppressive doses of prednisone (tapered over a 9-month period, with no evidence of disease off prednisone over the next 8 months of follow-up), and one dog was in complete remission and was on month 7 of tapering immunosuppressive doses of prednisone. The second dog was treated with 2 months of a tapering immunosuppressive dose of prednisone and improved. This dog relapsed 1 month after prednisone was discontinued, but when prednisone was reinstituted, the dog "did well" for 4 months before developing acute respiratory distress and neurologic signs (euthanasia was performed, but no postmortem examination was allowed). The cat with BOOP had waxing and waning

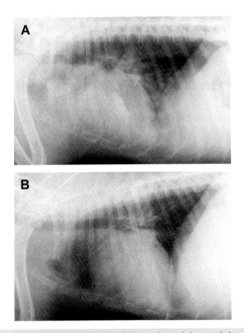

Fig. 1. (A) Lateral radiograph of a 1.5-year-old large-breed dog with histologically confirmed bronchiolitis obliterans with organizing pneumonia. Nodular interstitial and coalescing alveolar infiltrates are noted, particularly in the cranial and ventral lung regions. (B) Lateral radiograph from the same dog after 7 days of treatment with prednisone at a dose of 2 mg/kg shows dramatic clearing of pulmonary infiltrates.

clinical signs for 18 months before being lost to follow-up. It would seem that the prognosis is good for dogs with naturally developing BOOP that respond to immunosuppressive doses of glucocorticoids; however, disease may relapse if glucocorticoids are tapered too rapidly. Although many cases are likely to be idiopathic, for cases with an underlying trigger (eg, inhalation of toxic fumes; drug reaction; viral, mycoplasmal, bacterial, or fungal infections), addressing the predisposing cause is likely to result in the most beneficial outcome.

PAP has only been described in two dogs to date [9,10]. As has been described in human beings, a series of therapeutic large-volume bronchoalveolar lavage (spaced 6 months apart) was used successfully to dilute and remove the lipoproteinaceous material from the lungs in one of these dogs [9,10]. This treatment would need to be tried in additional dogs with PAP before strong conclusions could be made. The use of GM-CSF in human patients with PAP holds promise, but this therapy has not been evaluated in dogs to date [37].

SUMMARY
Several noninfectious nonneoplastic ILDs have been recognized in dogs and cats, including eosinophilic pneumonia, IPF, LIP, BOOP, EnLP, PAP, silicosis, and asbestosis. Overall, these ILDs are poorly characterized in dogs and cats,

although awareness of the conditions based on descriptions of clinical case series may be increasing. Lung biopsy remains crucial to the diagnosis, characterization, and classification of ILDs. Histopathologic findings can help to guide clinicians in selecting appropriate therapy and providing an accurate prognosis to pet owners. Only with definitive recognition of these pulmonary conditions can our knowledge of the clinical course and response to therapy be improved.

References

[1] Norris C, Mellema M. Eosinophilic pneumonia. In: King L, editor. Textbook of respiratory diseases in dogs and cats. Philadelphia: WB Saunders Co; 2004. p. 541–7.

[2] Lobetti R, Milner R, Lane E. Chronic idiopathic pulmonary fibrosis in five dogs. J Am Anim Hosp Assoc 2001;37:119–27.

[3] Cadore J, Steiner-Laurent S, Greenland T, et al. Interstitial lung disease in feline immunodeficiency virus (FIV) infected cats. Res Vet Sci 1997;62:287–8.

[4] Phillips S, Barr S, Dykes N, et al. Bronchiolitis obliterans with organizing pneumonia in a dog. J Vet Intern Med 2000;14:204–7.

[5] Canfield P, Rothwell T, Padpdimitriou J, et al. Siliceous pneumoconiosis in two dogs. J Comp Pathol 1989;89:199–202.

[6] Schuster N. Pulmonary asbestosis in a dog. J Pathol Bacteriol 1931;34:751–7.

[7] Jerram R, Guyer C, Braniecki A, et al. Endogenous lipid (cholesterol) pneumonia associated with a bronchogenic carcinoma in a cat. J Am Anim Hosp Assoc 1998;34:275–80.

[8] Raya AI, Fernandez-de Marco M, Nunez A, et al. Endogenous lipid pneumonia in a dog. J Comp Pathol 2006;135:153–5.

[9] Jefferies A, Dunn J, Dennis R. Pulmonary alveolar proteinosis (phospholipoproteinosis) in a dog. J Small Anim Pract 1987;28:203–14.

[10] Silverstein D, Greene C, Gregory C, et al. Pulmonary alveolar proteinosis in a dog. J Vet Intern Med 2000;14:546–51.

[11] Clercx C, Peeters D, Snaps F, et al. Eosinophilic bronchopneumopathy in dogs. J Vet Intern Med 2000;14:282–91.

[12] Cohn L, Norris C, Hawkins E, et al. Identification and characterization of an idiopathic fibrosis-like condition in cats. J Vet Intern Med 2004;18:632–41.

[13] Corcoran B, Cobb M, Martin M, et al. Chronic pulmonary disease in Welsh Highland white terriers. Vet Rec 1999;144:611–6.

[14] Norris C, Griffey S, Walsh P. Use of keyhole lung biopsy for diagnosis of interstitial lung diseases in dogs and cats: 13 cases (1998–2001). J Am Vet Med Assoc 2002;221:1453–9.

[15] Jones D, Norris C, Samii V, et al. Endogenous lipid pneumonia in cats: 24 cases (1985–1998). J Am Vet Med Assoc 2000;216:1437–40.

[16] Li X, Botts S, Morton D, et al. Oleic acid-associated bronchiolitis obliterans-organizing pneumonia in beagle dogs. Vet Pathol 2006;43:183–5.

[17] Quigley M, Hansell D, Nicholson A. Interstitial lung disease—the new synergy between radiology and pathology. Histopathology 2006;49:334–42.

[18] Calvert C, Mahaffey M, Lappin M, et al. Pulmonary and disseminated eosinophilic granulomatosis in dogs. J Am Anim Hosp Assoc 1987;24:311–20.

[19] Lord P, Schaer M, Tilley L. Pulmonary infiltrates with eosinophilia in the dog. J Amer Vet Radiol Soc 1975;16:115–20.

[20] Moon M. Pulmonary infiltrates with eosinophilia. J Small Anim Pract 1992;33:19–23.

[21] Noone K. Pulmonary hypersensitivities. In: Kirk RW, editor. Current veterinary therapy IX. Philadelphia: WB Saunders; 1986. p. 285–92.

[22] Sykes JE, Weiss DJ, Buoen LC, et al. Idiopathic hypereosinophilic syndrome in 3 Rottweilers. J Vet Intern Med 2001;15:162–6.

[23] Williams K, Malarkey D, Cohn L, et al. Identification of spontaneous feline idiopathic pulmonary fibrosis: morphology and ultrastructural evidence for a type II pneumocyte defect. Chest 2004;125:2278–88.

[24] Corcoran B, Dukes-McEwan J, Rhind S, et al. Idiopathic pulmonary fibrosis in a Staffordshire bull terrier with hypothyroidism. J Small Anim Pract 1990;40:185–8.

[25] Rhind S, Gunn-Moore D. Desquamative form of cryptogenic fibrosing alveolitis in a cat. J Comp Pathol 2000;123:226–9.

[26] Norris A, Naydan D, Wilson D. Interstitial lung disease in West Highland white terriers. Vet Pathol 2005;42:35–41.

[27] Dempsey O. Clinical review: idiopathic pulmonary fibrosis—past, present and future. Respir Med 2006;100:1871–85.

[28] Kirchner B, Port C, Magoc T, et al. Spontaneous bronchopneumonia in laboratory dogs infected with untyped Mycoplasma spp. Lab Anim Sci 1990;40:625–8.

[29] Castleman W. Bronchiolitis obliterans and pneumonia induced in young dogs by experimental adenovirus infection. Am J Pathol 1985;119:495–504.

[30] Dungworth D. The respiratory system. In: Jubb KFV, Kennedy PC, Palmer N, editors. Pathology of domestic animals. 4th edition. San Deigo (CA): Academic Press; 1993. p. 610–3.

[31] King T, et al. Interstitial lung diseases. In: Braunwald E, Fauci AS, Kasper DL, editors. Harrison's principles of internal medicine. 15th edition. New York: McGraw Hill; 2001. p. 1499–513.

[32] Schwartz L, Knight H, Whittig L, et al. Silicate pneumoconiosis and pulmonary fibrosis in horses from the Monterey-Carmel Peninsula. Chest 1981;80:82S–5S.

[33] Johnson V, Corcoran B, Wotton P, et al. Thoracic high-resolution computed tomographic findings in dogs with canine idiopathic pulmonary fibrosis. J Small Anim Pract 2005;46:381–8.

[34] Schechter J, Norris C, Griffey S, et al. Correlation between fine-needle aspiration cytology and histology of the lung in dogs and cats. J Am Anim Hosp, in press.

[35] DeBerry JD, Norris C, Griffey S, et al. Correlation between fine-needle aspiration cytopathology and histopathology of the kung in dogs and cats. J Anim Hosp 2002;38(4):327–36.

[36] Norris C, Griffey S, Samii V, et al. Thoracic radiography, bronchoalveolar cytology, and pulmonary parenchymal histology: a comparison of diagnostic results in 11 cats. J Am Anim Hosp 2002;38:337–45.

[37] Ioachimescu O, Kavuru M. Pulmonary alveolar proteinosis. Chron Respir Dis 2006;3:149–59.

Cardiac Effects of Pulmonary Disease

Fiona E. Campbell, BVSc (Hons), MACVSc, PhD[a,b,*]

[a]Veterinary Medical Teaching Hospital, School of Veterinary Medicine, University of California, Davis at Davis, CA, USA
[b]Veterinary Teaching Hospital, School of Veterinary Science, University of Queensland, 95 Chermside Road, St. Lucia, Queensland 4305, Australia

Pulmonary hypertension (PHT), the primary cardiac consequence of pulmonary disease, is most frequently described in the veterinary literature as single case reports and a few case series [1–10]. The exception is PHT secondary to heartworm disease, which has been studied extensively and is largely excluded from this review. PHT is a deleterious sequela of pulmonary disease, and severe PHT confers a grave prognosis. Screening for PHT in at-risk patients with respiratory disease may facilitate instigation of specific therapies, which, although unproven, are aimed at attenuating PHT and its clinical consequences while also providing valuable prognostic information for the attending veterinarian and dog owner.

PATHOPHYSIOLOGY OF PULMONARY HYPERTENSION SECONDARY TO PULMONARY DISEASE

The most common pulmonary cause of PHT in people is chronic obstructive pulmonary disease [11]. In dogs, many respiratory diseases, including pneumonia, tracheobronchial disease, infiltrative pulmonary disease, laryngeal paralysis, pulmonary thromboembolism, *Angiostrongylus vasorum* infestation, interstitial pulmonary fibrosis of West Highland White Terriers, neoplasia, and *Dirofilaria immitis*, have been reported to produce PHT, with *D immitis* infestation being most common in heartworm-endemic regions [1,4–6,8,12].

The pathophysiology of PHT is multifactorial and can largely be attributed to an increase in pulmonary vascular resistance resulting from vasoconstriction and vascular remodeling in response to regional and perfusional hypoxemia and release of endogenous vasoactive mediators and mitogens from diseased pulmonary endothelial and smooth muscle cells, activated platelets, and inflammatory cells [13]. Vascular remodeling, characterized by medial hypertrophy and intimal fibrosis [14], and vasoconstriction reduce arterial luminal

*Veterinary Teaching Hospital, School of Veterinary Science, University of Queensland, 95 Chermside Road, St. Lucia, Queensland 4305, Australia.
E-mail address: f.campbell@uq.edu.au

0195-5616/07/$ – see front matter
doi:10.1016/j.cvsm.2007.05.006

dimension and pulmonary compliance, and the reduction in total cross-sectional area of the pulmonary arterial bed results in an increase in pulmonary vascular resistance. In patients with underlying pulmonary disease, the vascular area may be further reduced by extraluminal (compressive) and intraluminal (obstructive) pathologic conditions [15]. Compensatory polycythemia in dogs with chronic hypoxemia (PaO_2 <45 mm Hg) [16] secondary to severe respiratory disease may exacerbate elevated pulmonary vascular resistance and PHT, because the increase in red blood cell concentration confers an exponential increase in blood viscosity [17].

Hypoxia uniquely elicits a well-recognized adaptive vasoconstrictor response in the pulmonary vascular bed that facilitates shunting of blood to better ventilated regions of the lung to improve ventilation-perfusion mismatching in patients with focal alveolar hypoxia [18]. This physiologic mechanism contributes to the development of PHT when pulmonary hypoxia is chronic or global, however. The degree of pulmonary arterial vasoconstriction in response to hypoxia varies between and within species, and dogs are generally accepted to have low pulmonary vascular reactivity [19]. Recent studies demonstrate that healthy dogs living at altitude with chronic hypoxemia (mean PaO_2 of 52 mm Hg) develop only mild to moderate PHT with systolic pulmonary artery pressure estimated by means of Doppler echocardiography of between 34 and 55 mm Hg [20]. In addition to hypoxic-induced pulmonary vasoconstriction, hypoxia contributes to the development of PHT by stimulating vascular remodeling by means of platelet-derived growth factor and renin-angiotensin-aldosterone activation [11].

Endothelial cells and vascular smooth muscle cells damaged by primary pulmonary pathologic conditions as well as inflammatory cells and platelets attracted to the diseased lung are a source of growth factors and substances that promote vasoconstriction and vascular remodeling to result in PHT. Endothelial injury can retard production of vasodilatory substances, including nitric oxide, prostacyclin, and endothelial-relaxing factor, and enhance release of vasoconstrictors, such as endothelin (ET) [21]. ET, normally produced by pulmonary endothelial cells, elicits powerful vasoconstriction by means of the ETA receptor on vascular smooth muscle cells and vasodilation by means of the ETB receptor on endothelial and smooth muscle cells and induces proliferation of multiple cell types, including vascular smooth muscle [22]. Vascular pathologic change disrupts ET homeostasis, increases circulating ET levels, and upregulates and modifies ETB receptors to augment pulmonary vasoconstriction and vascular remodeling. The role of ET in the pathophysiology of PHT is supported by the clinical benefit of ET receptor blockers in patients with PHT [23,24]. Platelets may also contribute to the development of PHT through release of several mediators of vasoconstriction, including thromboxane, histamine, and serotonin [25]. Serotonin is a potent pulmonary vasoconstrictor and mitogen for pulmonary smooth muscle, and its role in the pathophysiology of PHT is demonstrated by the development of PHT in experimental animals with overexpression of serotonin transporters [26].

EFFECTS OF PULMONARY HYPERTENSION

Exercise intolerance is the most frequently observed clinical sign in dogs with PHT [8]. It occurs with PHT independent of exercise limitations imposed by the primary pulmonary disease because of ventilation-perfusion mismatching, lactic acidosis at a low work rate, arterial hypoxemia [27], and the inability of the right heart to increase pulmonary blood flow adequately through the fixed and noncompliant pulmonary vascular bed to meet the increased cardiac output demands of exercise [28].

Syncope occurs in more than 20% of dogs with PHT [8] and may be similarly attributable to inadequate pulmonary blood flow with exercise. Alternatively, syncope may occur as a result of vagally mediated reflex bradycardia and hypotension when an exercise-associated rise in right ventricular (RV) systolic pressure stimulates ventricular pressure receptors [29]. It is also possible that syncope may be attributable to ischemic-induced ventricular tachycardia in dogs with severe PHT, in which coronary perfusion is compromised by suprasystemic RV systolic pressures and the circumferential compressive stress associated with diastolic septal flattening [30].

Respiratory distress, tachypnea, and hyperpnea occur with PHT independent of precipitating pulmonary disease because of reduced lung compliance associated with vascular remodeling and hypoxemia of exertion [27].

Cor pulmonale is the term used to describe right-sided congestive heart failure that develops as a result of moderate to severe PHT [11]. Elevated pulmonary vascular resistance increases RV afterload, and compensatory RV hypertrophy develops to counter the increase in wall stress. When the hypertrophic capacity of the right ventricle is exceeded, or if the increase in pulmonary vascular resistance occurs acutely before the right ventricle has time to hypertrophy (eg, pulmonary thromboembolism), diastolic ventricular pressure rises. This elevation in diastolic ventricular pressure is exacerbated if secondary RV myocardial failure develops or if hemodynamically significant tricuspid regurgitation occurs secondary to ventricular dilation and expansion of the tricuspid annulus. Right atrial distention and contractility increase to maintain RV filling [31], but once the compensatory capacity of the right atrium (RA) is overwhelmed, systemic venous pressures rise sufficiently to produce signs of right-sided heart failure.

DIAGNOSIS OF PULMONARY HYPERTENSION

Physical examination reveals increased respiratory rate and effort attributable to the primary pulmonary disease and secondary PHT. Thoracic auscultation is abnormal, and the distribution and severity of pulmonary crackles and wheezes reflect the underlying pulmonary pathologic condition. Cardiac auscultation may be unremarkable or may reveal a low-grade right-sided systolic murmur of tricuspid regurgitation [2,5,8] or, rarely, a low-grade left basilar diastolic murmur of pulmonic insufficiency or a split second heart sound. Turbulent blood flow sufficient to produce a palpable thrill should not occur with the degree of valvular insufficiency produced by annular dilation associated with

PHT, and its presence is indicative of concurrent primary cardiac disease. Premature beats and associated pulse deficits occasionally occur in patients with severe PHT in the absence of primary cardiac disease [5]. Pulse quality is usually normal, except in extremely severely affected dogs in which pulmonary vascular resistance is sufficient to limit pulmonary blood flow, reduce venous return to the left ventricle, and decrease systemic blood flow [3,5]. Cyanosis may be present depending on the severity of the primary pulmonary disease and manifests more readily in chronically hypoxic patients with compensatory polycythemia [32]. Signs of systemic congestion and edema, including jugular venous distention, hepatomegaly, and ascites, may be identified in dogs with severe PHT and cor pulmonale.

Thoracic radiographs provide essential information in the diagnosis and severity assessment of primary pulmonary disease but are insensitive for the identification of PHT. Radiographs of dogs with severe PHT may demonstrate dilation of the cranial and caudal lobar pulmonary arteries, although except for heartworm disease, in which pulmonary artery changes may be profound, pulmonary artery dilation is subtle in most cases. Caudal lobar pulmonary arteries may not exceed previously reported normal limits in which comparison is made between the arteries and the width of the ninth rib at their point of intersection [33], but their relative dilation may be appreciated by comparison with the smaller paired vein. In severe cases of PHT, dilation of the main pulmonary artery may be identified as a bulge at the 1- to 2-o'clock position on the cardiac silhouette on the dorsoventral radiograph. Right heart enlargement may also be identified by increased sternal contact of the heart on the lateral projection, together with a reverse-D shape of the cardiac silhouette on the dorsoventral film [33]. Care should be taken in interpreting right heart enlargement from the lateral film alone, because tachypnea associated with pulmonary disease may preclude acquisition of an image at full inspiration and cardiac sternal contact may be accentuated. Systemic congestion and edema secondary to severe PHT may be evident, including caudal vena caval dilation, pleural effusion, hepatomegaly, and ascites (Fig. 1).

In addition to evaluating the effects of pulmonary disease on the heart, thoracic radiographs facilitate exclusion of cardiogenic causes of respiratory signs. With the rare exception of acute volume overload attributable to mitral valve chordae tendineae rupture or endocarditis of the aortic or mitral valve, normal left atrial size is indicative of a left ventricular diastolic pressure that is normal and insufficient to cause pulmonary venous congestion and cardiogenic pulmonary edema. The nature and distribution of pulmonary infiltrates may also support exclusion of cardiogenic pulmonary edema as the cause for respiratory distress.

Echocardiography is the test of choice for the diagnosis of PHT in veterinary patients with pulmonary disease. Two-dimensional and m-mode echocardiography often demonstrate abnormalities suggestive of PHT. The acquired pressure load conferred by moderate to severe PHT results in a combination of eccentric and concentric hypertrophy of the right ventricle, observed on

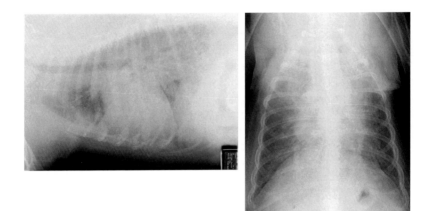

Fig. 1. Right lateral and dorsoventral and thoracic radiographs of an 11-year-old female spayed Giant Schnauzer with severe PHT (systolic pulmonary artery pressure estimated by Doppler echocardiography of 85 mm Hg) and cor pulmonale secondary to chronic pulmonary disease. The caudal lobar pulmonary arteries are enlarged, trivial pleural effusion is present, and despite limited capacity to interpret pulmonary parenchyma in the presence of pleural effusion, a diffuse heavy interstitial and peribronchial pattern is evident. Although this patient had RV concentric and eccentric hypertrophy and RA dilation identified echocardiographically, these cannot be appreciated radiographically. The increased cardiac sternal contact apparent on the lateral film may be attributable to shallow chest conformation and the expiratory phase of the respiratory cycle at which the film was acquired rather than to right heart enlargement. Pleural effusion obscures assessment of the cardiac silhouette on the dorsoventral projection.

two-dimensional echocardiography as ventricular dilation and increased RV wall thickness, respectively [8]. Identification of normal pulmonic valve structure and mobility, together with laminar pulmonary flow of normal velocity, is important to exclude pulmonic stenosis as the cause of increased RV afterload. In dogs with severe PHT, dilation of the main pulmonary artery and a pulmonary artery root–to–aortic root ratio of greater than 1 are often observed. Flattening of the interventricular septum during systole occurs with severe PHT when systolic pulmonary artery pressure exceeds systemic systolic arterial pressure, and diastolic interventricular septal flattening occurs in patients with cor pulmonale when diastolic pressure of the right ventricle exceeds that of the left ventricle. A reduction in left ventricular diastolic dimension may also be observed and reflects the reduction in venous return to the left heart in dogs when severe PHT limits pulmonary blood flow [2,6,8].

Doppler echocardiography allows definitive diagnosis and quantification of PHT in patients with tricuspid regurgitation or pulmonic insufficiency [34]. Low-velocity trivial tricuspid regurgitation, which is hemodynamically insignificant and inaudible, can be detected in 30% to 80% of healthy dogs [12,35]. Tricuspid regurgitation is discovered with a similar or higher frequency in dogs with PHT [12,20,35], and the velocity of regurgitation determines the magnitude of PHT. Application of the modified Bernoulli equation (4 × [velocity in meters per second]^2) to the tricuspid regurgitant flow velocity assessed by continuous-wave Doppler echocardiography allows determination of an RV-to-RA pressure gradient during ventricular systole. In the absence of pulmonic stenosis, RV and pulmonary artery pressures are equal, such that systolic pulmonary artery pressure can be estimated by addition of the RV-to-RA pressure gradient to the assumed pressure of the RA (Fig. 2). Likewise, diastolic pulmonary artery pressure can be estimated in patients with pulmonic insufficiency by the addition of the pressure gradient between the pulmonary artery and right ventricle, derived from pulmonic insufficiency flow velocity, to the assumed RA pressure. Estimated systolic pulmonary artery pressure is most frequently used to classify the PHT as mild (30–55 mm Hg), moderate (55–80 mm Hg), or severe (>80 mm Hg) [5].

The diagnostic value of other echocardiographically derived variables has been evaluated in veterinary patients with PHT. Systolic time intervals of pulmonary artery flow in dogs with PHT secondary to pulmonary disease or heartworm disease demonstrate a reduction in acceleration time and acceleration time to ejection time ratio, and the sensitivity and specificity of this method may be sufficient for definitive diagnosis of PHT in dogs that lack tricuspid or pulmonic insufficiency [12,36]. Increased pulsed-wave Doppler mitral inflow A-wave velocity, reduced E-to-A wave ratio, reduced left ventricular pre-ejection period (LVPEP), and shortened LVPEP-to–ejection time ratio have been identified in dogs with PHT, but the low sensitivity and specificity of these variables preclude their usefulness in diagnosis of PHT [37].

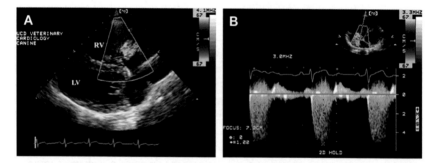

Fig. 2. (A) Color-flow Doppler echocardiography of a right parasternal long-axis image of the heart of a 4-year-old female spayed Border Collie with severe PHT demonstrating RV dilation (eccentric hypertrophy), increased RV wall thickness (concentric hypertrophy), RA dilation, and tricuspid regurgitation. (B) Continuous wave Doppler assessment of the tricuspid regurgitant flow demonstrates increased flow velocity of 4.5 m/s, from which an RV-to-RA pressure gradient of 81 mm Hg is calculated using the modified Bernoulli equation. RA pressure was assumed to be 10 mm Hg because of signs of systemic congestion, including hepatic and jugular venous dilation and ascites, resulting in an estimated systolic pulmonary artery pressure of 91 mm Hg.

There are several limitations to the echocardiographic diagnosis of PHT. Pulmonary disease that requires mechanical ventilation or is associated with overinflated or emphysematous lungs compromises the quality of the acoustic window necessary for echocardiographic examination. Severe trepopnea may prevent examination of the patient in lateral recumbency. Suboptimal patient positioning may preclude acquisition or result in nonparallel alignment of the Doppler beam with subsequent underestimation of trivial tricuspid or pulmonic insufficiency flow velocity [34]. Echocardiography can be insensitive at detecting mild and mild to moderate PHT [35] or acute PHT secondary to pulmonary thromboembolism [38] in which the two-dimensional and m-mode examination is normal. Lack of changes suggestive of PHT on routine echocardiography increases the importance of Doppler-derived tricuspid or pulmonic regurgitant flow velocity for identification of PHT, yet the absence of tricuspid or pulmonic insufficiency occurs in approximately 20% of human patients with catheter-confirmed PHT [39]. Another limitation of echocardiographic diagnosis of PHT is the assumption of RA pressure. Generally, a RA pressure of 5 mm Hg is assumed in the absence of systemic congestion and edema, and a RA pressure of 10 mm Hg is assumed in patients with systemic congestive signs [5]. The error in this assumption is most relevant to patients with mild PHT, in which a 5- to 10-mm Hg discrepancy may significantly alter the estimated pulmonary artery pressure when added to the low RV-to-RA or RV-to–pulmonary artery pressure gradient. Because reference ranges of pulmonary artery pressures in conscious healthy dogs are not well defined, assessment of dogs with mild to moderate PHT is also confounded [40]. In dogs, PHT determined noninvasively by Doppler echocardiographic estimation of pulmonary artery pressure is variably defined as systolic pulmonary artery pressure exceeding 30 mm Hg [5], 35 mm Hg [8,20,35], or 45 mm Hg [12]. In human patients, pulmonary artery pressure is influenced by age, gender, body mass index, and athletic level [27,41]. Whether the same is true for dogs has not been investigated, and additional factors unique to veterinary patients, including breed, thoracic conformation, and neuter status, may also confound defined normal limits of pulmonary artery pressure.

Because it allows direct measurement of pulmonary artery pressures and, in association with thermodilution-derived cardiac output, facilitates calculation of pulmonary vascular resistance, cardiac catheterization is the "gold standard" for diagnosis of PHT [27]. In human patients, diagnostic cardiac catheterization also allows assessment of acute vasoreactivity to short-acting vasodilators and identification of candidates for chronic oral vasodilator therapy [27]. Cardiac catheterization is rarely performed in dogs with suspected PHT, because general anesthesia is often necessary in veterinary patients, which reduces pulmonary artery pressures and may be associated with significant morbidity and mortality of dogs with pulmonary disease. Moreover, Doppler echocardiography is a valid surrogate, and studies in people demonstrate close correlation between Doppler estimated and directly measured pulmonary artery pressures [39].

ECG can provide suggestive or supportive evidence of PHT by demonstrating morphologic changes associated with RV hypertrophy and RA dilation [2,5,8,10], but it lacks the sensitivity and specificity to be used as a screening tool [42]. Arrhythmia detection on physical examination warrants an ECG examination, because increased RV afterload poses a risk for ischemic-related ventricular arrhythmias [30]; the author and others [5] have identified ventricular arrhythmias in dogs with PHT.

TREATMENT OF PULMONARY HYPERTENSION

Treatment of underlying pulmonary disease is fundamental in dogs with secondary PHT. With the exception of heartworm disease, however, inciting pulmonary disease sufficient to cause PHT is often severe and irreversible. Specific treatment (eg, antibiotics for bacterial pneumonia) and nonspecific therapeutics (eg, weight loss to improve tidal volume and related alveolar hypoxia in obese patients) should be used, with the aim of attenuating or reversing primary pulmonary pathologic change.

A secondary aim of treatment is to lower pulmonary artery pressure to limit or delay the clinical sequelae of PHT by reducing the pulmonary vasoconstriction and vascular remodeling that mediate increased pulmonary vascular resistance. Traditionally, the candidacy of human patients with PHT for chronic vasodilator therapy is assessed by means of cardiac catheterization by response to short-acting vasodilators [25,43]. Subsequent long-term calcium channel blocker or continuous intravenous prostacyclin therapy improves quality of life and survival of vasoreactivity-tested responders with primary PHT [25,44–46]; however, these vasodilators are less than ideal, because a central venous line is required for continuous prostacyclin infusion. Also, each therapy lacks pulmonary smooth muscle selectivity and has the propensity to cause systemic hypotension and reflex tachycardia, which may compromise coronary perfusion [25]. Other therapeutics used in human patients with PHT include oxygen therapy; oral anticoagulants [47]; inhaled nitric oxide [48]; oral, subcutaneous, and inhaled prostacyclin analogues [49–51]; endothelin receptor antagonists [22–24]; atrial septostomy; and lung transplantation [52].

Case reports of dogs with primary and secondary PHT describe the use of some of these vasodilator agents [2,3,5], but a lack of controlled studies precludes assessment of drug efficacy in veterinary patients. Any theoretic benefit of vasodilators in dogs with PHT may be limited by the low pulmonary vasoreactivity in this species [19]. Also, use of vasodilator agents in dogs with PHT secondary to respiratory disease could instead exacerbate ventilation-perfusion mismatch by interfering with the physiologic hypoxic vasoconstrictor mechanism and dilating nonventilated regions of the lung [53].

Recently, the phosphodiesterase-5 (PDE-5) inhibitor sildenafil (Viagra) has been investigated to treat PHT. PDE-5 is abundant in pulmonary vascular smooth muscle, and enzyme levels are upregulated in PHT [54]. Inhibition of PDE-5 elevates cyclic guanine monophosphate, which opens specific potassium channels and selectively vasodilates pulmonary arteries [54]. Interestingly, oral sildenafil administered to human patients with PHT secondary to pulmonary fibrosis selectively dilated well-ventilated regions of the lung and improved ventilation-perfusion matching [53]. Sildenafil also seems to attenuate vascular remodeling by cyclic guanine monophosphate–mediated suppression of transcription factors for smooth muscle cell production of serine vascular elastase [55–57]. The frequency of ventricular arrhythmias in dogs with PHT is unknown, but the ability of sildenafil to attenuate ventricular tachycardia might also be beneficial [58]. Sildenafil may have additional benefits in dogs with PHT secondary to airway disease through reduction of airway hyperreactivity and leukocyte chemotaxis [59].

Randomized, double-blind, placebo-controlled trials of sildenafil in human patients with primary and secondary PHT have demonstrated improved quality of life and exercise capacity [55,60]. Furthermore, a clinical benefit was demonstrated in patients who failed traditional invasive vasoreactivity testing [56]. A retrospective report of 13 dogs with PHT of unknown cause (n = 8) or secondary to pulmonary disease (n = 5) described a reduction in systolic pulmonary artery pressure estimated by Doppler echocardiographic measurement of tricuspid regurgitant flow velocity and an improvement of clinical signs [9]. Anecdotally, the author's experience has been similar to that reported by Bach and colleagues [9], whereby the addition of sildenafil to treatments for underlying pulmonary disease produces a moderate reduction in Doppler estimated pulmonary artery pressure and some alleviation of clinical signs in most dogs, although these apparent benefits are not sustained long term (Fig. 3). Prospective randomized controlled trials are clearly needed to identify any statistically significant benefit of sildenafil. Studies are also required to determine the optimal dose of sildenafil for dogs. The half-life of sildenafil is only a few hours [54], and a wide range of dosage regimens have been used in dogs, from as little as 0.5 mg/kg every 24 hours [9] up to 6 mg/kg every 4 hours [5]. The longer acting PDE-5 inhibitor tadanafil may also show promise for treatment of dogs with PHT [7].

Treatment of systemic congestion and edema is warranted in dogs with cor pulmonale that are not sufficiently palliated by therapeutics aimed at underlying pulmonary disease or resultant PHT. Diuretics and abdominocentesis can be used, but care should be taken to avoid unnecessarily aggressive diuresis that may reduce venous return and compromise cardiac output. Angiotensin-converting enzyme inhibitors have not been successful in reducing pulmonary artery pressure in hypoxia-induced pulmonary vasoconstriction [61]; however, because the renin-angiotensin-aldosterone system is activated in human patients with PHT [25] and in dogs with cor pulmonale [62], their use may be warranted.

PROGNOSIS OF PULMONARY HYPERTENSION

The prognosis of human patients with PHT is related to the severity of the PHT and the underlying respiratory disease [27]. With the exception of heartworm disease, respiratory disease sufficient to result in PHT in dogs is almost

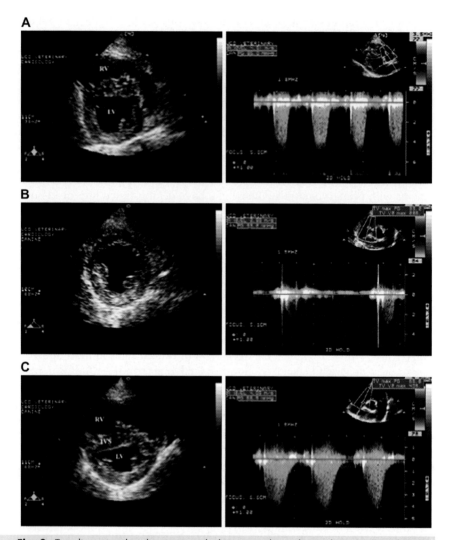

Fig. 3. Two-dimensional, right parasternal, short-axis echocardiographic images and continuous-wave Doppler flow profiles of tricuspid regurgitation from the 11-year-old female spayed Giant Schnauzer with severe PHT described in Fig. 1. (A) Initial diagnostic echocardiogram identified an estimated systolic pulmonary artery pressure of 85 mm Hg. (B) Subsequent examination after 5 months of treatment for underlying respiratory disease and use of sildenafil showed a reduction in estimated systolic pulmonary artery pressure (38 mm Hg) and reversal of the compensatory RV changes. (C) Repeated examination 10 months after initial diagnosis identified recurrence of moderate to severe PHT (estimated systolic pulmonary artery pressure of 77 mm Hg) and RV concentric and eccentric hypertrophy. Notice the flattening of the interventricular septum (IVS) during diastole at initial and final examination, indicating that RV pressure exceeds left ventricular diastolic pressure and is sufficient to produce signs of systemic congestion.

universally irreversible and fatal [2,3,5,6,8–10]. Because survival times are confounded by the nature of primary pulmonary disease and elective euthanasia, reported median survival times of dogs with PHT of 3 days [8] and 91 days [9] are of limited clinical application, except to emphasize the grave prognosis of PHT associated with respiratory disease. It follows that these studies, unlike those in human beings, failed to find prognostic value in the degree of PHT estimated by Doppler echocardiography [8,9]. The recent application of PDE-5 inhibitors for the treatment of PHT shows promise for palliation of dogs with PHT secondary to respiratory disease [9], but the prognosis should remain guarded at best.

SUMMARY

The effects of pulmonary disease on the heart are directed by the development of PHT. Alveolar hypoxia of respiratory disease, coupled with vasoactive and mitogenic substances released from endothelial and vascular smooth muscle cells damaged by the primary pulmonary disease process, mediates arterial vasoconstriction and vascular remodeling. In turn, pulmonary arterial compliance and total cross-sectional area of the pulmonary arterial bed are reduced, raising pulmonary vascular resistance and resulting in PHT. PHT increases afterload on the right ventricle and, independent of underlying pulmonary disease, produces respiratory signs, syncope, and right heart failure. Severe PHT, irrespective of the inciting pulmonary cause, confers a grave prognosis.

References

[1] Estaves I, Tessier D, Dandrieux J, et al. Reversible pulmonary hypertension presenting simultaneously with an atrial septal defect and angiostrongylosis in a dog. J Small Anim Pract 2004;45(4):206–9.

[2] Glaus TM, Soldati G, Maurer R, et al. Clinical and pathological characterisation of primary pulmonary hypertension in a dog. Vet Rec 2004;154:786–9.

[3] Kolm US, Amberger CN, Boujon CE, et al. Plexogenic pulmonary arteriopathy in a Pembroke Welsh corgi. J Small Anim Pract 2004;45:461–6.

[4] Nicolle AP, Chetboul V, Tessier-Vetzel D, et al. Severe pulmonary arterial hypertension due to Angiostrongylus vasorum in a dog. Can Vet J 2006;47(8):792–5.

[5] Pyle RL, Abbott JA, MacLean HN. Severe pulmonary hypertension and cardiovascular sequelae in dogs. Vet Med 2004;99(6):530–41.

[6] Pyle RL, King MD, Saunders GK, et al. Pulmonary thrombosis due to idiopathic main pulmonary artery disease. Vet Med 2004;99(10):836–42.

[7] Serres F, Nicolle AP, Tissier R, et al. Efficacy of oral tadalafil, a new long-acting phosphodiesterase-5 inhibitor, for short-term treatment of pulmonary arterial hypertension in a dog. J Vet Med A Physiol Pathol Clin Med 2006;53(3):129–33.

[8] Johnson LR, Boon JA, Orton EC. Clinical characteristics of 53 dogs with Doppler-derived evidence of pulmonary hypertension: 1992–1996. J Vet Intern Med 1999;13:440–7.

[9] Bach JF, Rozanski EA, MacGregor J, et al. Retrospective evaluation of sildenafil citrate as a therapy for pulmonary hypertension in dogs. J Vet Intern Med 2006;20:1132–5.

[10] Brewster RD, Benjamin SA, Thomassen RW. Spontaneous cor pulmonale in laboratory beagles. Lab Anim Sci 1983;33(3):299–302.

[11] McLaughlin VV, Rich S. Cor pulmonale. In: Baunwald E, Zipes DP, Libby P, editors. Heart disease: a textbook of cardiovascular medicine. 6th edition. Philadelphia: WB Saunders; 2001. p. 1936–54.

[12] Schober KE, Baade H. Doppler echocardiographic prediction of pulmonary hypertension in West Highland White Terriers with chronic pulmonary disease. J Vet Intern Med 2006;20: 912–20.

[13] Voelkel NF, Tuder RM. Cellular and molecular mechanisms in the pathogenesis of pulmonary hypertension. Eur Respir J 1995;8:2129–38.

[14] Pietra GG, Capron F, Stewart S, et al. Pathologic assessment of vasculopathies in pulmonary hypertension. J Am Coll Cardiol 2004;43:25S–32S.

[15] Perry LA, Dillon AR, Bowers T. Pulmonary hypertension. The Compendium on Continuing Education for the Practicing Veterinarian 1991;13(2):226–32.

[16] Kittleson MD, Kienle RD. Patent ductus arteriosus. In: Kittleson MD, Kienle RD, editors. Small animal cardiovascular medicine. New York: Mosby; 1998. p. 218–30.

[17] Pirofsky B. The determination of blood viscosity in man by a method based on Poiseuille's law. J Clin Invest 1953;32:292–8.

[18] Ganong WF. Pulmonary function. In: Foltin J, Mattagrano M, Ranson J, et al, editors. Review of medical physiology. East Norwalk (CT): Appleton and Lange; 1995. p. 591–607.

[19] Wauthy P, Pagnamenta A, Vassalli F, et al. Right ventricular adaptation to pulmonary hypertension: an interspecies comparison. Am J Physiol Heart Circ Physiol 2004;286(4): H1441–7.

[20] Glaus TM, Hassig M, Baumgartner C, et al. Pulmonary hypertension induced in dogs by hypoxia at different high-altitude levels. Vet Res Commun 2003;27:661–70.

[21] Budhiraja R, Tuder RM, Hassoun PM. Endothelial dysfunction in pulmonary hypertension. Circulation 2004;109:159–65.

[22] Channick RN, Sitbon O, Barst RJ, et al. Endothelin receptor antagonists in pulmonary arterial hypertension. J Am Coll Cardiol 2004;43(12):62S–7S.

[23] Channick RN, Simonneau G, Sitbon O, et al. Effects of the dual endothelin-receptor antagonist bosentan in patients with pulmonary hypertension: a randomised placebo-controlled study. Lancet 2001;358:1119–23.

[24] Rubin LJ, Badesch D, Barst RJ, et al. Bosentan therapy for pulmonary arterial hypertension. N Eng J Med 2002;346:896–903.

[25] Archer S, Rich S. Primary pulmonary hypertension. Circulation 2000;102:2781–91.

[26] Eickelberg O, Yeager ME, Grimminger F. The tantalizing triplet of pulmonary hypertension-BMP receptors, serotonin receptors and angiopoietins. Circ Res 2003;60:465–7.

[27] Barst RJ, McGoon MD, Torbicki A, et al. Diagnosis and differential assessment of pulmonary arterial hypertension. J Am Coll Cardiol 2004;43(12):40S–7S.

[28] Hoeper MM, Oudiz RJ, Peacock A, et al. End points and clinical trial designs in pulmonary arterial hypertension. J Am Coll Cardiol 2004;43(12):48S–55S.

[29] Zucker IH, Cornish KG. The Bezold-Jarisch reflex in the conscious dog. Circ Res 1981;49: 940–8.

[30] Nelson GS, Sayed-Ahmed EY, Kroeker CA, et al. Compression of interventricular septum during right ventricular pressure loading. Am J Physiol Heart Circ Physiol 2001;280(6): H2639–48.

[31] Gaynor SL, Maniar HS, Bloch JB, et al. Right atrial and ventricular adaptation to chronic right ventricular pressure overload. Circulation 2005;112(9):I212–8.

[32] Kittleson MD. Signalment, history and physical examination. In: Kittleson MD, Kienle RD, editors. Small animal cardiovascular medicine. New York: Mosby; 1998. p. 36–46.

[33] Thrall DE. Textbook of veterinary diagnostic radiology. 3rd edition. Philadelphia: Saunders; 1998.

[34] Boon JA. Manual of veterinary echocardiography. Baltimore (MD): Williams and Wilkins; 1998.

[35] Glaus TM, Hauser K, Hassig M, et al. Non-invasive measurement of the cardiovascular effects of chronic hypoxaemia on dogs living at moderately high altitude. Vet Rec 2003;152:800–3.

[36] Uehara Y. An attempt to estimate the pulmonary artery pressure in dogs by means of pulsed Doppler echocardiography. J Vet Med Sci 1993;55:307–12.

[37] Glaus TM, Tomsa K, Hassig M, et al. Echocardiographic changes induced by moderate to marked hypobaric hypoxia in dogs. Vet Radiol Ultrasound 2004;45(3):233–7.

[38] Johnson LR, Michael MR, Baker DC. Pulmonary thromboembolism in 29 dogs: 1985–1995. J Vet Intern Med 1999;13:338–45.

[39] Currie PJ, Seward JB, Chan KL, et al. Continuous wave Doppler determination of right ventricular pressure: a simultaneous Doppler-catheterization study in 127 patients. J Am Coll Cardiol 1985;6:750–6.

[40] Gross DR. Normal cardiovascular parameters from intact, awake animals. In: Gross DR, editor. Animal models in cardiovascular research. Boston: Kluwer; 1994. p. 343–95.

[41] McQuillan BM, Picard MH, Leavitt M, et al. Clinical correlates and reference intervals for pulmonary artery systolic pressure among echocardiographically normal subjects. Circulation 2001;104:2797–802.

[42] Ahearn GS, Tapson VF, Rebeiz A, et al. Electrocardiography to define clinical status in primary pulmonary hypertension and pulmonary arterial hypertension secondary to collagen vascular disease. Chest 2002;122:524–7.

[43] Dunbar I. Diagnosis and treatment of severe pediatric pulmonary hypertension. Cardiol Rev 2001;9(4):227–36.

[44] Barst RJ, Rubin LJ, Long WA. A comparison of continuous intravenous epoprostenol (prostacyclin) with conventional therapy for primary pulmonary hypertension. The Primary Pulmonary Hypertension Study Group. N Engl J Med 1996;30(334):296–302.

[45] Higenbottam T, Wells F, Wheeldon D, et al. Long-term treatment of primary pulmonary hypertension with continuous intravenous epoprostenol (prostacyclin). Lancet 1984;1:1046–7.

[46] Rich S, Kaufmann E, Levy PS. The effect of high doses of calcium-channel blockers on survival in primary pulmonary hypertension. N Eng J Med 1992;327:76–81.

[47] Fuster V, Steele PM, Edwards WD, et al. Primary pulmonary hypertension: natural history and importance of thrombosis. Circulation 1984;70:580–7.

[48] Ivy DD, Parker D, Doran A, et al. Acute hemodynamic effects and home therapy using a novel pulsed nasal nitric oxide delivery system in children and young adults with pulmonary hypertension. Am J Cardiol 2003;92:886–90.

[49] Badesch D, McLaughlin VV, Delcroix M, et al. Prostanoid therapy for pulmonary arterial hypertension. J Am Coll Cardiol 2004;43(12):56S–61S.

[50] Mikhail G, Gibbs JSR, Richardson M, et al. An evaluation of nebulized prostacyclin in patients with primary and secondary pulmonary hypertension. Eur Heart J 1997;18:1499–504.

[51] Olschewski H, Simonneau G, Galie N, et al. Inhaled iloprost for severe pulmonary hypertension. N Eng J Med 2002;347:322–9.

[52] Klepetko W, Mayer E, Sandoval J, et al. Interventional and surgical modalities of treatment for pulmonary arterial hypertension. J Am Coll Cardiol 2004;43(12):73S–80S.

[53] Ghofrani HA, Pepki-Zaba J, Barbera JA, et al. Nitric oxide pathway and phosphodiesterase inhibitors in pulmonary arterial hypertension. J Am Coll Cardiol 2004;43(12):68S–72S.

[54] Wright PJ. Comparison of phosphodiesterase type 5 inhibitors. Int J Clin Pract 2006;60(8):967–75.

[55] Galie N, Ghorani HA, Torbicki A, et al. Sildenafil citrate therapy for pulmonary arterial hypertension. N Eng J Med 2005;352(20):2148–57.

[56] Humpl T, Reyes JT, Holtby H, et al. Beneficial effect of oral sildenafil therapy on childhood pulmonary arterial hypertension. Circulation 2005;111:3274–80.

[57] Mitani Y, Zaidi SH, Dufourcq P, et al. Nitric oxide reduces vascular smooth muscle cell elastase activity through cGMP-mediated suppression of ERK phosphorylation and AML1B nuclear partitioning. FASEB J 2000;14:805–14.

[58] Nagy O, Hagnal A, Parratt JR, et al. Sildenafil reduces arrhythmia severity during ischemia 24 h after oral administration in dogs. Br J Pharmacol 2004;141(4):549–51.

[59] Toward TJ, Smith N, Broadley KJ. Effect of phosphodiesterase-5 inhibitor, sildenafil, in animal models of airway disease. Am J Respir Crit Care Med 2004;169(2):227–34.

[60] Sastry BK, Narasimhan C, Reddy NK, et al. Clinical efficacy of sildenafil in primary pulmonary hypertension. J Am Coll Cardiol 2004;43:1149–53.

[61] Hubloue I, Rondelet B, Kerbaul F, et al. Endogenous angiotensin II in the regulation of hypoxic pulmonary vasoconstriction in anesthetized dogs. Crit Care 2004;8(4):R163–71.

[62] Buoro IBJ, Atwell RB. Plasma levels of renin and aldosterone in right-sided congestive heart failure due to canine dirofilariasis. Canine Pract 1992;17(3):21–4.

Advances in Respiratory Therapy

Elizabeth A. Rozanski, DVM[a],*, Jonathan F. Bach, DVM[b],
Scott P. Shaw, DVM[a]

[a]Section of Critical Care, Department of Clinical Sciences, Cummings School of Veterinary Medicine, Tufts University, 200 Westboro Road, North Grafton, MA 01536, USA
[b]Department of Medical Sciences, University of Wisconsin School of Veterinary Medicine, 2015 Linden Drive, Madison, WI 53706, USA

Therapy in pulmonology, as in all subspecialties, is most effective when a specific recognized therapy is available for a precise diagnosis. For example, it is more rewarding to treat an *Escherichia coli* pneumonia susceptible to enrofloxacin than it is to treat a "chronic snuffling sound, with a little clear nasal discharge" in a dog. Many respiratory diseases can be effectively treated or cured with antibiotics, anti-inflammatory agents, or chemotherapeutic drugs; however, chronic inflammatory diseases and those with undefined causes remain difficult to manage. As in all fields, advancing knowledge may lead to improved outcome and quality of life. Recent advances in pulmonary therapeutics can be divided into new pharmaceutics (drugs) and new methods of drug delivery.

NEW PHARMACEUTICS

Use of new drugs and development of new applications for established drugs are common in veterinary medicine. The astute clinician should recognize that the best use of a new drug follows positive results from at least a single if not multiple placebo-controlled double-blind studies. That said, use of most drugs in veterinary medicine does not follow those guidelines; thus, the decision to use or not to use a drug in a specific patient should be based on careful evaluation of the risk-to-benefit ratio, objective monitoring, and informed client consent. In some cases, different but closely related drugs may have different efficacies. It is also important to remember that cats have unique metabolic pathways that influence efficacy and toxicity.

Recent additions to the respiratory armamentarium include the fluoroquinolones, azithromycin (Zitromax), sildenafil (Viagra), and leukotriene receptor antagonists. Additionally, the pharmacokinetic properties of theophylline have recently been re-evaluated in dogs and in cats, and the use of doxapram for evaluation of laryngeal function has been incorporated into the mainstream

*Corresponding author. E-mail address: elizabeth.rozanski@tufts.edu (E.A. Rozanski).

0195-5616/07/$ – see front matter
doi:10.1016/j.cvsm.2007.05.009

[1–3]. Finally, in cats with experimentally created asthma, rush immunotherapy has been explored as a therapeutic option [4].

Fluoroquinolones

The fluoroquinolone class of antibiotics was originally introduced in the late 1980s with the prototypical drugs ciprofloxacin and enrofloxacin (Baytril). Since that time, several other fluoroquinolones have been introduced for the veterinary market, including difloxacin (Dicural), marbofloxacin (Zeniquin), and orbifloxacin (Orbax). The mechanism of action is primarily by inhibition of bacterial replication through an effect on DNA gyrase. Interestingly, similar to the penicillins, the activity of fluoroquinolones is bacteriostatic at low doses, although at therapeutic doses, it is bactericidal [5]. At extremely high doses, bactericidal activity may actually be impaired, perhaps because of inhibition of protein synthesis [5]. Fluoroquinolones are particularly appealing for use in respiratory disease for many reasons, including excellent penetration into the respiratory system, accumulation in the epithelial lining fluid and in macrophages, and a broad spectrum of activity against most gram-negative organisms and *Mycoplasma*. As a rule, fluoroquinolones are not effective in vivo against *Streptococcus* species or against anaerobes. Therefore, before obtaining sensitivity data on a sample, a fluoroquinolone should be combined with another antibiotic, such as amoxicillin, to achieve broad-spectrum coverage. Additionally, when evaluating bacterial sensitivity data, the actual fluoroquinolone intended for use should be evaluated, because despite similar mechanisms of action, variations in sensitivities exist [6]. Generic ciprofloxacin has recently become available and may represent a significant cost savings to patients being treated long term, although the bioavailability of ciprofloxacin in veterinary patients is far less than that of enrofloxacin. As of this writing (December 2006), at the Tufts Cummings School of Veterinary Medicine, a 250-mg tablet of generic ciprofloxacin costs $0.17 per tablet, whereas a 136-mg tablet of enrofloxacin is $2.39, a 100-mg tablet of marbofloxacin is $2.67, and a 68-mg tablet of orbifloxacin is $3.59.

An important consideration for the clinical use of fluoroquinolones includes the recognized side effects of the drug class, including blindness, which has been reported in cats in association with use of enrofloxacin, and the potential for abnormalities associated with cartilage in growing animals. Importantly, fluoroquinolones, like most antimicrobials, have poor penetration into tracheal and bronchial secretions. Consequently, systemic use for kennel cough complex does not hasten resolution of disease and may contribute to bacterial resistance. Finally, in respiratory patients in particular, if theophylline is administered in conjunction with ciprofloxacin or enrofloxacin, the metabolism of theophylline (a methylxanthine) is decreased, which may potentially lead to toxicity by increasing plasma theophylline concentration.

Azithromycin

Azithromycin has gained popularity over the past decade as a respiratory antibiotic [7]. It should be noted that azithromycin is generally grouped with the macrolide class of antibiotics because it shares many of the properties of a macrolide, although it is technically an azalide [7]. Macrolides represent a large group of similar compounds that are products of *Streptomyces* spp. Biochemically, they are characterized by a macrocyclic lactone ring attached to one or more sugar moieties. Macrolides with the greatest clinical efficacy are generally derived from erythromycin.

Azithromycin acts by reversibly binding to the 50S ribosome [7] and suppressing RNA-dependent protein synthesis. Azithromycin is bacteriostatic at clinical concentrations. It is particularly effective against gram-positive organisms and *Mycoplasma* spp, although it has some activity against gram-negative organisms as well. In addition, it has fair efficacy against anaerobic organisms.

Azithromycin is stable in acid and, as a result, has high oral bioavailability [7]. Azithromycin seems to be rapidly taken up by tissues and then slowly released. Tissue concentrations are generally 10 to 100 times those achieved in serum, and the drug can be concentrated 200 to 500 times in macrophages. This high level of drug in macrophages may not always be advantageous because it can suppress phagocytic activity. Azithromycin does not exhibit any effect on gastrointestinal smooth muscle; as a result, gastrointestinal side effects are uncommon.

Azithromycin is commonly used by veterinarians to treat severe respiratory infections. It can be highly effective in resolving chronic persistent pneumonia, particularly that secondary to *Bordetella* infection [8]. Care should be taken when using azithromycin as a sole agent because of the limitations of its gram-negative spectrum and the fact that resistance is a growing problem. In addition, one study found azithromycin to be ineffective in clearing chlamydophilosis in a clinical trial, although clinical signs were improved [9]. Azithromycin is commonly administered at 5 to 10 mg/kg once a day for 5 to 7 days, although other schemes exist as well.

Sildenafil

Pulmonary hypertension (PHT) is a devastating condition in dogs that is typically associated with a poor outcome [10]. Sildenafil (Viagra), which was first introduced into human medicine as therapy for erectile dysfunction (ED), has been shown to be useful in reducing pulmonary artery pressure and decreasing clinical signs in people and dogs with PHT [11,12]. Sildenafil is a phosphodiesterase (PDE) type V inhibitor that results in increased concentrations of cyclic guanosine monophosphate (GMP) in vascular smooth muscle cells and subsequent nitric oxide–mediated vasodilation of the pulmonary vasculature. A recent retrospective study reported on the use of sildenafil in 13 dogs with naturally occurring PHT [11]. This report described mild to moderate improvements in pulmonary arterial pressures and quality of life after addition of sildenafil as therapy. Further studies are needed to validate this finding and to determine an optimal dosing strategy. The published dose is 0.5 mg to 2.7 mg/kg every 8 to 24 hours. The authors start sildenafil therapy at approximately 1 mg/kg administered orally every 8 hours and titrate upward if needed. Sildenafil therapy can result in systemic hypotension and must not be combined with nitrates, such as nitroglycerin, or profound hypotension may result. Sildenafil is marketed as an oral PHT therapy under the trade name of Revatio in 20-mg tablets. Because one of the main limitations to widespread use of sildenafil is its high cost, however, it is much more cost-effective to divide 100 mg tablets of Viagra for use in veterinary patients. A longer acting PDE-5 inhibitor (tadalafil) might prove useful in therapy. Other oral ED drugs, such as vardenafil (Levitra), are only now being evaluated in people with PHT but may ultimately be useful in dogs as well [13].

Leukotriene Receptor Antagonists

Although prednisone remains the primary therapy for airway inflammation in human asthmatic patients, the high rate of side effects associated with chronic therapy has led to development of alternative modulators of inflammation, including leukotriene receptor antagonists, such as zafirlukast (Accolate) and montelukast (Singulair). The only controlled study in the literature that examined the role of leukotriene blockers was performed in cats with experimentally created asthma and found no benefit to therapy with zafirlukast [14]. Therefore, such therapy is not likely to be effective, although additional studies are perhaps needed in naturally affected cats. In a small blind study of dogs with atopy, zafirlukast was beneficial in 11% (2 of 18) of dogs, which actually compared favorably with the clinical response to commonly used antihistamines [15]. The role, if any, of leukotriene receptor antagonists remains to be determined in veterinary pulmonology.

Extended-Release Theophylline

Theophylline is a methylxanthine, similar to caffeine, and this drug has been widely used in respiratory medicine as a bronchodilator. The specific mechanism of action responsible for bronchodilatory properties seems to be multifactorial [1]. Theophylline is a nonspecific phosphodiesterase inhibitor and may lead to bronchodilation by means of increased concentrations of cyclic adenosine monophosphate (cAMP). Theophylline also acts as an antagonist of adenosine, one of the proposed mediators involved in asthma. Theophylline has nonspecific effects, such as decreasing diaphragmatic fatigue and increasing mucociliary clearance (in dogs), that may result in clinical improvement in respiratory patients.

It is well established that various extended-release formulations of theophylline available in human pharmacies do not result in similar plasma concentrations [16]. Pharmacokinetic studies had established dosages for products available in 2001; however, these drugs were withdrawn from the market, and re-evaluation of bioavailability and pharmacokinetics of currently available products was required. In a recent study, dogs that were dosed at 10 mg/kg orally every 12 hours using the product manufactured by Inwood Laboratories, Inc. (Commack, New York) developed plasma theophylline concentrations within the therapeutic range described for human beings [1]. In cats, using the same Inwood Laboratories, Inc. product, a dose of 15 mg/kg for the tablets and 19 mg/kg for the capsules administered orally once daily was found to provide an acceptable plasma concentration [3]. Previously, evening administration of theophylline has been recommended in cats because of improved chronopharmacokinetics.

Doxapram

Doxapram hydrochloride (Dopram-V) is a centrally acting respiratory stimulant. Doxapram's original clinical use was for the treatment of apnea or hypoventilation, although intubation and manual ventilation are far more effective and should supersede the use of doxapram for these conditions. In 2002, Miller and colleagues [2] introduced the use of doxapram into clinical medicine for evaluation of laryngeal dysfunction. In small animals, laryngeal examination requires sedation, and although some agents have more or less effect on intrinsic motion, in all cases, the examiner may be confounded by the degree of sedation required to visualize the larynx (Fig. 1) [17]. Doxapram is administered intravenously at a dose of 1 mg/lb (2.2 mg/kg), and the observed effect is almost immediate in animals with normal laryngeal function, with an increase in opening of the rima glottis. Tobias and colleagues [18] validated the utility of doxapram hydrochloride for detecting laryngeal paralysis in 2004.

Rush Immunotherapy

Rush immunotherapy is a technique pioneered 50 years ago by which an individual is rapidly hyposensitized to a specific allergen over a period of hours to days rather than over the more typical period of weeks to months. The appeal of rush immunotherapy is the opportunity to cure the individual of an allergy within a short time [19]. Rush immunotherapy is particularly popular for desensitizing individuals with severe insect (eg, bee and wasp) allergies [20]. Rush immunotherapy was evaluated in a group of cats with experimentally induced asthma by Reinero and colleagues [4]. This study documented a decrease in eosinophilic airway inflammation in treated cats compared with untreated cats, and relatively few side effects were encountered. The current limitation of rush immunotherapy in cats is the lack of knowledge or ability to identify a specific allergen responsible for the syndrome of feline asthma.

Intraluminal Tracheal Stents

Tracheal collapse is a progressive degenerative condition that most often affects middle-aged to older toy and miniature breed dogs. Medical management has included antitussives, anxiolytics, avoiding neck leashes, weight loss, and, occasionally, corticosteroids. Surgical options have used extraluminal polypropylene stabilization for dogs with cervical tracheal collapse. Recently the use of self-expanding intraluminal stents has gained further acceptance, and success has been shown in alleviating life-threatening clinical signs associated with airway obstruction and unrelenting cough [21]. Placement of such stents requires specialized equipment (eg, fluoroscopy, tracheoscopy). Complications, including stent migration, pneumothorax, stent compression, and infection, seem to

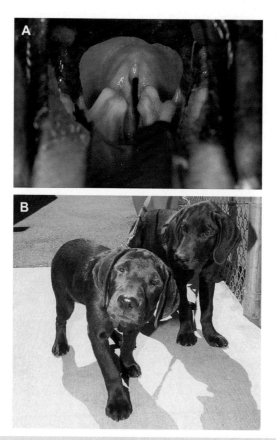

Fig. 1. An excellent knowledge of normal anatomy and function of the larynx is required for the pulmonologist. (A) Image illustrates the larynx of a Labrador Retriever puppy affected with congenital laryngeal paralysis. (B) This defect, which was associated with a progressive neurodegenerative disorder, was also accompanied by microphthalmia.

occur less frequently with the newer products that are specifically measured for the individual dog and with increased familiarity with the procedure [22].

Propofol

Finally, no discussion of advances in respiratory therapy would be complete without mention of the anesthetic agent propofol. The widespread availability and overall safety profile of propofol have led to increased opportunities to perform short invasive respiratory procedures and transoral tracheal aspirates in patients with respiratory compromise. It is crucial to remember that the use of propofol is not without risk, because apnea and hypotension are often seen with its use, similar to thiopental. The most appealing characteristics of propofol are its rapid metabolic rate and limited period of recovery, which makes it clinically useful for outpatient procedures and for rapid recovery of inpatients.

NEW METHODS OF DRUG DELIVERY
The two major novel methods of pulmonary drug delivery include aerosol therapy for parenchymal and lower airway disease and intracavitary therapy for pleural space diseases.

Aerosol Therapy
Aerosol therapy is commonly used in human medicine to provide local delivery of a variety of medications to the airways. Aerosol therapy has also been used with good success in horses [23,24]. Because of equipment challenges and an inherent lack of cooperation in companion animals, aerosols have not been widely used in cats or dogs. Recently, however, there has been renewed interest and enthusiasm for the development of face mask equipment for use in the dog and cat. The two companies that have been the most proactive in the field of small animal aerosol therapy are Trudell Medical (London, Ontario, Canada) [25] and IVX Animal Health (Fort Dodge, Iowa).

To understand aerosol therapy, it is important to review the technical aspects of aerosol delivery and the normal physical response to particulate inhalation. Deposition of aerosol particles within the respiratory tract depends on their size as well as on the patient's tidal volume, inspiratory flow rate, and ability to breath hold. Optimal particle size for delivery to the trachea is 2 to 10 μm and is 0.5 to 5 μm in the peripheral airways. Particle size depends on the type of nebulizer or metered dose inhaler (MDI) used. In dogs and cats, aerosols are usually delivered by means of an ultrasonic or compressed air nebulizer. The drug to be nebulized is placed within a medication cup, and the nebulizer unit is connected to a baffle that generates the particles. The patient is typically placed within a cage or carrier and receives the nebulization treatment for a specific length of time. It is important to differentiate a medical-grade nebulizer from a "humidifier" that merely generates water vapor.

Aerosol therapy is considered desirable as a method of drug delivery to limit systemic absorption and to direct therapy at the site of the problem. Diseases that are considered particularly amenable to aerosol therapy include feline lower airway disease, canine chronic bronchitis, and kennel cough complex in puppies [26]. Aerosol treatment with a bronchodilator has also been used as a preventive therapy against bronchoconstriction during bronchoscopic bronchoalveolar lavage. A study in cats with experimentally induced lower airway disease documented a beneficial effect of pretreatment with an aerosolized bronchodilator in preventing bronchoconstriction associated with the lavage procedure [27].

Agents that are considered potentially beneficial when administered by means of the aerosol route include physiologic saline; some antibiotics (particularly aminoglycosides); glucocorticoids (through commercially available MDIs); and bronchodilators, including β_2 agonists, such as albuterol, and anticholinergics, such as ipratropium [28]. Doses that are currently recommended for use in veterinary patients are somewhat arbitrary, because human dosing is based on cooperation with instructions to inhale deeply and to momentarily hold one's breath.

Feline bronchitis is a common airway disease with clinical signs that range from mild and intermittent to severe and life threatening. Most cats respond extremely well to oral anti-inflammatory treatment with prednisone or prednisolone, and some clinicians advocate concurrent use of oral bronchodilators, such as theophylline or terbutaline. Aerosol therapy has been proposed as a method for limiting complications of systemic glucocorticoids by local treatment with inhaled glucocorticoids or use of an inhaled β_2 agonist for immediate relief of bronchoconstriction. Rational initial treatment of asthmatic cats should be directed at controlling the crisis with oral or injectable glucocorticoids before considering a transition to inhaled glucocorticoids. It is prudent to warn clients that inhaled glucocorticoids are expensive ($100 every 1–2 months), particularly when contrasted with the costs associated with oral prednisolone. Some cats do well with intermittent treatment with an inhaled β_2 agonist during a crisis; however, it is not appropriate to treat cats with inhaled β_2 agonists on a regular basis because this approach has been shown to increase the likelihood of complications in people as a result of uncontrolled and progressive airway inflammation. Most cats do tolerate inhaled therapy, particularly in a home environment, but some cats are quite challenging to treat.

Canine chronic bronchitis is another common inflammatory airway disease that responds well to oral prednisone. Infection may occasionally complicate chronic bronchitis as well as tracheal collapse [29], and dogs with acute flare-up of disease may benefit from the addition of oral antibiotics. Because the presence of infection is a relative contraindication to the use of oral prednisone, addition of inhaled steroids may be useful in these instances. Although dogs are more intrinsically cooperative than cats, they may resent application of the face mask and aerosol spacer, and this may lead to treatment failure. Dogs have not been documented to experience bronchoconstriction in association with chronic bronchitis, and a benefit for aerosolized bronchodilators has not been established. Eosinophilic bronchopneumopathy is a second inflammatory disease of the airways and lung parenchyma that may be controlled with the use of inhaled steroids. Because affected dogs often require long-term steroid therapy, inhaled drugs can be beneficial in limiting systemic side effects.

Kennel cough complex is common in puppies, particularly those from "puppy mills." Most cases of kennel cough are rapidly self-limiting; however, some severely affected puppies may benefit from nebulized antibiotics in addition to systemic therapy for pneumonia. Aminoglycosides are particularly amenable to delivery by nebulization, and this treatment modality can hasten recovery from infection as well as limit the potential for side effects from systemic administration, such as nephrotoxicity. A recent abstract documented the clinical utility of this treatment for affected puppies in clinical practice [26].

Addition of aerosolized or nebulized drugs into the therapeutic regimen for the pet with respiratory disease can aid in control of clinical signs and reduce systemic side effects. The use of nebulized aminoglycosides for kennel cough complex and inhaled steroids for treatment of chronic inflammatory airway disease is particularly exciting. Use of other medications should be considered adjuvant to conventional therapy rather than as a replacement for systemic medications.

Intracavitary Therapy

Pleural effusion represents a common clinical condition in cats and dogs. In most cases, the underlying cause of the effusion can be rapidly determined and treated. A malignant pleural effusion may be primary, caused by pleural mesothelioma or other local neoplasms, or secondary to metastatic disease, most commonly, carcinoma. In human medicine, when malignant pleural effusion accompanies a lung mass, the tumor is often considered inoperable and the course of care may transition from curative to palliative. In people with lung cancer, identification of neoplastic pleural lavage cytology has been associated with a poor prognosis, and there is growing interest in the use of intraoperative pleural lavage to look for evidence of metastatic disease [30]. Therefore, the presence of a lung mass with malignant pleural effusion could be considered likely to represent metastatic disease in veterinary medicine, and it might be wise to pursue a course of therapy designed to control local disease.

Intracavitary therapy is pursued by infusing a chemotherapeutic agent directly into the pleural space. Local infusion of chemotherapy should be considered in animals with diffuse involvement of the pleural space. The chemotherapeutic agent is able to penetrate 1 to 3 mm into the pleura, thus exposing neoplastic cells to a high local concentration of drug. Cisplatin has been used most frequently for this purpose in dogs at a dose of 50 mg/m^2 every 3 to 6 weeks. Cisplatin is associated with renal toxicity; thus, a standard diuresis protocol should be employed before use. Intracavitary carboplatin (180–300 mg/m^2) has also been used in dogs and cats and has the advantage of not requiring diuresis before use as well as reduced gastrointestinal toxicity. Mitoxantrone has also been used at a dose of 5 to 5.5 mg/m^2. In a retrospective study of intracavitary chemotherapy of four dogs treated for malignant pleural effusion, survival times ranged from 18 days to 299 days after treatment with carboplatin or mitoxantrone [31].

The ultimate role of intracavitary chemotherapy remains to be determined, but it seems to be a viable option in some patients because it is associated with limited morbidity. Animals with rapid fluid reaccumulation may be much harder to manage because of dilution of the chemotherapeutic agent by pleural fluid. Technically, the procedure is performed as outlined in Fig. 2. Preexisting pleural effusion should be removed, and the chemotherapeutic agent should be slowly infused over several minutes. In small or compromised pets, thoracostomy tubes may be replaced by a butterfly catheter or an over-the-needle catheter. The patient should be rolled from side to side to assist with distribution of the agent throughout the thoracic cavity and then monitored for 5 to 15 minutes before discharge. In dogs with long-standing large-volume effusion (eg, 2–3 L), cough is commonly reported during the 24 hours after treatment. Reinfusion of chemotherapy may be pursued on an as-needed basis or every 4 to 6 weeks.

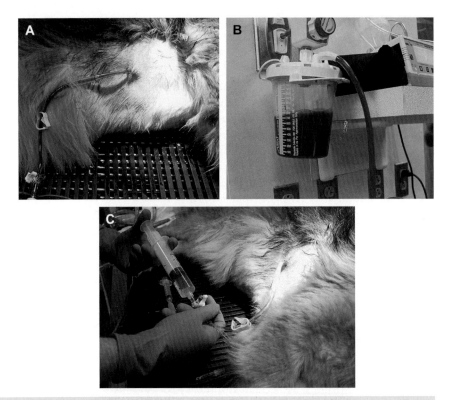

Fig. 2. Treatment of an intrathoracic malignancy can be achieved with intracavitary infusion of chemotherapeutic agents, including cisplatin or carboplatin. (*A, B*) Small-bore chest tube is placed for evacuation of fluid. (*C*) Chemotherapy agent is then infused, and the patient is rolled to help distribute the drug.

SUMMARY

Advances in pharmaceutics and in drug delivery have occurred over the past 10 to 15 years in veterinary pulmonology. Clinicians should look for evidence-based studies evaluating the efficacies of these newer therapies to help establish their role in clinical practice.

References

[1] Bach JE, Kukanich B, Papich MG, et al. Evaluation of the bioavailability and pharmacokinetics of two extended-release theophylline formulations in dogs. J Am Vet Med Assoc 2004;224:1113–9.

[2] Miller CJ, McKiernan BC, Pace J, et al. The effects of doxapram hydrochloride (Dopram-V) on laryngeal function in healthy dogs. J Vet Intern Med 2002;16:524–8.

[3] Guenther-Yenke CL, McKiernan BC, Papich MG, et al. Evaluation of the bioavailability and pharmacokinetics of an extended release theophylline product in cats. In: Proceedings of the 24th Symposium of the Veterinary Comparative Respiratory Society, Oct 2006, Jena, Germany. Available at: http://www.the-vcrs.org.

[4] Reinero CR, Byerly JR, Berhaus RD, et al. Rush immunotherapy in an experimental model of feline allergic asthma. Vet Immunol Immunopathol 2006;110:141–53.

[5] Martinez M, McDermott P, Walker R. Pharmacology of the fluoroquinolones: a perspective for the use in domestic animals. Vet J 2006;172:10–28.

[6] Riddle C, Lemons CL, Papich MG, et al. Evaluation of ciprofloxacin as a representative of veterinary fluoroquinolones in susceptibility testing. J Clin Microbiol 2001;39:1680–1.

[7] Hunter RP, Lynch MJ, Ericson JF, et al. Pharmacokinetics, oral bioavailability and tissue distribution of azithromycin in cats. J Vet Pharmacol Ther 1995;18:38–46.

[8] Papich MG, Bidgood T. Antimicrobial drug therapy. In: Ettinger SJ, Feldman EC, editors. Textbook of veterinary internal medicine. St Louis (MO): Elsevier-Saunders; 2005. p. 498–503.

[9] Owen WM, Sturgess CP, Harbour DA, et al. Efficacy of azithromycin for the treatment of feline chlamydophilosis. J Feline Med Surg 2003;5:305–11.

[10] Johnson L, Boon J, Orton EC. Clinical characteristics of 53 dogs with Doppler-derived evidence of pulmonary hypertension: 1992–1996. J Vet Intern Med 1999;13:440–7.

[11] Bach JF, Rozanski EA, MacGregor J, et al. Retrospective evaluation of sildenafil citrate as a therapy for pulmonary hypertension in dogs. J Vet Intern Med 2006;20:1132–5.

[12] Raja SG, Danton MD, MacArthur KJ, et al. Treatment of pulmonary arterial hypertension with sildenafil: from pathophysiology to clinical evidence. J Cardiothorac Vasc Anesth 2006;20:722–35.

[13] Aizawa K, Hanaoka T, Kasai H, et al. Long-term vardenafil therapy improves hemodynamics in patients with pulmonary hypertension. Hypertens Res 2006;29:123–8.

[14] Reinero CR, Decile KC, Byerly JR, et al. Effects of drug treatment on inflammation and hyperactivity of airways and on immune variables in cats with experimentally induced asthma. Am J Vet Res 2005;66:1121–7.

[15] Senter DA, Scott DW, Miller WH. Treatment of canine atopic dermatitis with zafirlukast, a leukotriene-receptor antagonist: a single-blinded, placebo-controlled study. Can Vet J 2002;43:203–6.

[16] Koritz GD, McKiernan BC, Neff-Davis CA, et al. Bioavailability of four slow-release theophylline formulations in the beagle dog. J Vet Pharmacol Ther 1986;9:293–302.

[17] Jackson AM, Tobias K, Long C, et al. Effects of various anesthetic agents on laryngeal motion during laryngoscopy in normal dogs. Vet Surg 2004;33:102–6.

[18] Tobias KM, Jackson AM, Harvey RC. Effects of doxapram HCl on laryngeal function of normal dogs and dogs with naturally occurring laryngeal paralysis. Vet Anaesth Analg 2004;31:258–63.

[19] Cox L. Accelerated immunotherapy schedules: review of efficacy and safety. Ann Allergy Asthma Immunol 2006;97:126–37.

[20] Pasaoglu G, Sin BA, Misirligil Z. Rush hymenoptera venom immunotherapy is efficacious and safe. J Investig Allergol Clin Immunol 2006;16:232–8.

[21] Moritz A, Schneider M, Bauer N. Management of advanced tracheal collapse in dogs using intraluminal self-expanding biliary wallstents. J Vet Intern Med 2004;18:31–42.

[22] Available at: http://www.infinitimedical.com. Accessed June 18, 2007.

[23] Derksen FJ, Olszewski MA, Robinson NE, et al. Aerosolized albuterol sulfate used as a bronchodilator in horses with recurrent airway obstruction. Am J Vet Res 1999;60: 689–93.

[24] Mazan MR, Hoffman AM, Kuehn H, et al. Effect of aerosolized albuterol sulfate on resting energy expenditure determined by use of open-flow indirect calorimetry in horses with recurrent airway obstruction. Am J Vet Res 2004;64:235–42.

[25] Available at: http://www.aerokat.com. Accessed December 28, 2006.

[26] Miller CJM, McKiernan BC, Hauser C, et al. Gentamicin aerosolization for the treatment of infectious tracheobronchitis. J Vet Intern Med 2003;17:386.

[27] Kirschvink N, Leemans J, Delvaux F, et al. Bronchodilators in bronchoscopy-induced airflow limitation in allergen-sensitized cats. J Vet Intern Med 2005;19:161–7.

[28] Kirschvink N, Leemans J, Delvaux F, et al. Inhaled fluticasone reduces bronchial responsiveness and airway inflammation in cats with mild chronic bronchitis. J Feline Med Surg 2006;8:45–54.

[29] Johnson LR, Fales WH. Clinical and microbiologic findings in dogs with bronchoscopically diagnosed tracheal collapse: 37 cases (1990–1995). J Am Vet Med Assoc 2001;219: 1247–50.

[30] Nakagawa T, Okumura N, Kakodo Y, et al. Clinical relevance of intraoperative pleural lavage cytology in non-small cell lung cancer. Ann Thorac Surg 2007;83:204–8.

[31] Charney SC, Bergman PJ, McKnight JA, et al. Evaluation of intracavitary mitoxantrone and carboplatin for treatment of carcinomatosis, sarcomatosis and mesothelioma, with or without malignant effusions: a retrospective of 12 cases (1997–2002). Veterinary Comparative Oncology 2005;3:171–81.

Medical and Surgical Management of Pyothorax

Catriona M. Macphail, DVM, PhD

Department of Clinical Sciences, College of Veterinary Medicine and Biomedical Sciences, Colorado State University, Fort Collins, CO 80523, USA

ANATOMY AND PATHOPHYSIOLOGY

The thoracic or pleural cavity is the potential space between the lungs, mediastinum, diaphragm, and thoracic wall. It is lined by the pleura, a serous membrane that can be classified by the particular structure it covers. Visceral pleura covers the lungs, whereas parietal pleura lines the rest of the thoracic cavity. The parietal pleura is further classified into costal, diaphragmatic, and mediastinal pleurae. Controversy exists as to whether the mediastinum in dogs and cats is complete or whether fenestrations allow free communication between the two sides of the thoracic cavity [1,2]. Unilateral infusion of saline results in bilateral distribution in experimental dogs; however, it is unclear if the mediastinum is truly fenestrated or just easily disrupted by effusion [3]. Lack of communication between the two sides of the thoracic cavity could also occur if the mediastinum is fenestrated, but it becomes plugged under inflammatory conditions [4,5]. There are isolated reports of unilateral effusion in dogs and cats [2,6,7]; however, bilateral effusions are the clinical norm.

A small amount of transudative fluid is normally contained within the pleural space. The purpose of this fluid is to allow structures to slide freely during respiration. The production and absorption of this fluid represent a continuous process controlled by Starling's forces [8,9]: hydrostatic pressure forces fluid out of the vasculature, oncotic pressure maintains fluid within the vasculature, and a relatively impermeable vascular membrane maintains a dry pleural surface. Pleural effusion develops when disease processes alter normal fluid dynamics. Inflammatory conditions that result in pyothorax cause increases in capillary permeability and obstruction of lymphatic drainage because of the release of chemical mediators. This results in an influx of fluid, protein, and cells into the pleural space. Bacteria can enter the pleural space from compromised lung parenchyma, trachea, bronchus, esophagus, or thoracic wall.

E-mail address: cmacphai@lamar.colostate.edu

0195-5616/07/$ – see front matter
doi:10.1016/j.cvsm.2007.05.012

ETIOLOGY

The cause of pyothorax cannot always be identified. In dogs, a definitive cause has been reported in only 4% to 14% of cases [10,11], whereas an underlying cause has been found in 40% to 67% of feline cases [6,12,13]. Suspected and reported etiologies in dogs include migrating foreign material, penetrating bite wounds, extension of bronchopneumonia, extension of discospondylitis, esophageal perforation, parasitic migration, hematogenous spread, or iatrogenic causes [5,11,14–17]. Grass awns and plant material are the most commonly implicated migrating foreign bodies, because there is an association of pyothorax with young hunting dogs (Fig. 1) [10]. Grass awns enter the mouth when the animal is breathing hard, and the material migrates down the respiratory tree, carrying normal oral cavity flora into the lower airways [13,18]. Retrograde movement out of the respiratory tract is not possible, because many inhaled grasses are barbed; active respiration causes further antegrade movement into the lung parenchyma.

Causes of pyothorax identified in cats include extension of aspiration pneumonia, rupture of a pulmonary abscess, parasitic migration, foreign body penetration from the esophagus or lung, or penetrating thoracic bite wounds [6,12,19]. It is widely believed that the most common route of infection is through penetrating bite wounds from other cats [13,20]. Organisms isolated in cases of feline pyothorax are similar to bacteria cultured from subcutaneous bite wound abscesses, which are also consistent with the normal bacterial flora of the feline oropharynx [20,21]. It has been shown that cats with pyothorax are 3.8 times more likely to live in a multicat household when compared with a control population [13]. A seasonal association has been found in cases of feline pyothorax, with cases more likely to occur in late summer or fall [13,20]. Again, this is believed to be attributable to increases in fighting and

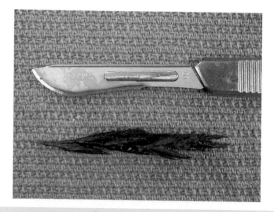

Fig. 1. Isolated grass awn removed from the lung of a 6-year-old male German Shorthaired Pointer with lung abscessation and pyothorax.

bite wounds in connection with warm weather and exposure to other cats [13]. It is theorized that these cats are more likely to incur penetrating thoracic bite wounds, although a supportive history or wound findings were only documented in 15% of cases and thoracic puncture wounds could be identified on necropsy in only 4 of 25 cats with pyothorax [13]. In contrast, other studies have theorized that the most common source of infection is aspiration of normal oropharyngeal flora and colonization of the lower respiratory tract [6]. Pyothorax then develops as an extension of infection from the lung into the pleural space, similar to what is described in human beings. The increased risk in multicat households could be as a result of greater exposure to upper respiratory viral infections, which may then predispose cats to bacterial pneumonia and resultant pyothorax [6,22].

Multiple bacterial organisms have been associated with pyothorax, but obligate anaerobes or a mixture of obligate anaerobes with facultative aerobic bacteria is the most common cause in dogs and cats [23]. *Pasteurella* spp are the most common organisms found in cats with pyothorax, whereas dogs have been associated with *Escherichia coli*; *Pasteurella* spp; and filamentous organisms, such as *Actinomyces* spp and *Nocardia* spp (Fig. 2). *Actinomyces* spp have been identified in 19% to 46% of dogs [11,23] and 10% to 15% of cats with pyothorax [6,13,23]. *Actinomyces* spp are most commonly associated with grass awn migration [15]. Other commonly identified organisms include *Bacteroides* spp, *Fusobacterium* spp, *Peptostreptococcus* spp, *Clostridium* spp, *Porphyromonas* spp, *Prevotella* spp, *Enterobacter* spp, *Klebsiella* spp, *Staphylococcus* spp, and *Streptococcus* spp [6,11,16,23,24]. Regional associations have also been identified, because suspected causes of pyothorax and organisms cultured differ between countries. For example, several European studies examined pyothorax in hunting breeds but found no evidence of migrating plant material as an underlying cause [17,25,26]. In contrast, plant material migration and *Actinomyces* spp infection are associated with hunting dogs in the United States [11,27].

DIAGNOSIS

The diagnosis of pyothorax in companion animals is usually straightforward and made from a combination of historic and physical examination findings, thoracic radiograph evaluation, and pleural fluid examination.

Signalment

The average age of onset of pyothorax is 4 to 5 years in dogs and cats, with ranges varying widely from several months of age to geriatric patients [6,10,11,13,23]. No overt breed predisposition has been identified, although the mean weight of dogs in one study was 25 kg [11]. Labrador Retrievers, Springer Spaniels, and Border Collies are the most common breeds reported [10,11,26,28]. For dogs and cats, male animals are overrepresented in numerous studies, although this finding has not been found to be statistically significant [6,10,11,13].

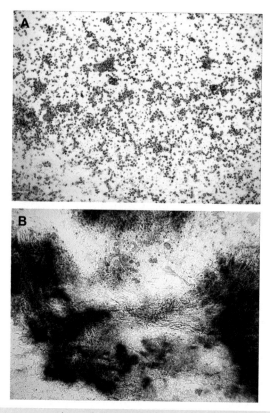

Fig. 2. (A) Inflammatory cytology of pleural fluid from a dog with pyothorax. (B) Multiple branching filamentous rods are noted consistent with *Actinomyces* spp or *Nocardia* spp infection.

Clinical Findings

Animals with pyothorax are expected to present with rapid shallow respirations indicative of a restrictive respiratory pattern attributable to fluid occupying the pleural space. Common clinical signs are nonspecific, however, and include lethargy, anorexia, weight loss, and coughing. In isolated reports, subcutaneous thoracic wall swellings have also been identified [23,25]. Approximately one third of cats with pyothorax demonstrate signs consistent with sepsis or systemic inflammatory response syndrome [13,16]. Other unique clinical signs that are associated with poor outcome in cats include bradycardia and hypersalivation [13]. The duration of clinical signs varies widely from days to months, and animals may present in acute distress or with more insidious signs of chronicity.

Hematologic and Biochemical Evaluation

Common hematologic findings include anemia and inflammatory leukograms. No association between the degree of leukocytosis and prognosis has been demonstrated in dogs [11]. In one study of feline pyothorax, however, cats that survived had a significantly higher white blood cell count than those that died [13]. It was theorized that lower neutrophil counts in nonsurviving cats were attributable to more severe pleural disease and sequestration of neutrophils in the pleural space or were secondary to severe sepsis. Biochemical abnormalities in dogs and cats with pyothorax are common but nonspecific. The most common abnormalities are hypoalbuminemia, hyperglobulinemia, hypo- or hyperglycemia, serum electrolyte imbalances, and mild elevations in serum liver enzyme activities [10,11,13].

Thoracic Radiographs
If an animal is severely compromised, thoracic radiographs should be delayed in favor of therapeutic thoracocentesis. Thoracic radiographs should ultimately be performed to assess the degree of pleural effusion, determine unilateral versus bilateral involvement, and evaluate for pulmonary or mediastinal masses. The appearance of pleural effusion on thoracic radiographs depends on the volume, character, and distribution of the fluid. Small amounts of fluid are best appreciated on a lateral thoracic view as soft tissue opacities that form wedges between the sternum and interlobar fissures of the lungs. These wedges may coalesce to give a scalloped appearance to the lung borders. There also tends to be blunting of the costophrenic angles. Classic roentgen signs of pleural effusion are seen when large amounts of pleural fluid are present, resulting in blurring of the cardiac silhouette and diaphragmatic border, the appearance of a widened mediastinum, and collapse of lung lobes (Fig. 3). Collapsed lung fields result in an alveolar pattern that can indicate atelectasis or pneumonia. Survey radiographs should be closely examined for possible underlying causes of pyothorax, such as mediastinal or pulmonary masses, pneumothorax, or pneumomediastinum.

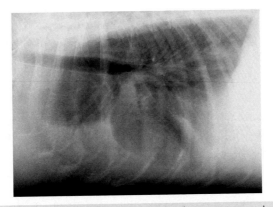

Fig. 3. Lateral thoracic radiograph of a dog with moderate to severe pleural effusion. The fluid obscures the cardiac silhouette and ventral diaphragmatic border.

Thoracic radiographs are also used to determine the quality of thoracostomy tube placement as well as to determine the effectiveness of the chosen therapy.

Pleural Fluid Analysis

Simple needle thoracocentesis is performed to obtain a fluid sample. Pleural fluid consistent with pyothorax is typically opaque and flocculent and can be hemorrhagic and malodorous. Diagnosis of a septic exudate is made when the protein concentration is greater than 3.0 g/dL, specific gravity is greater than 1.025, nucleated cell count is greater than 3000 cells/μL (although counts are often >30,000 cells/μL) with the predominant cell type being degenerate neutrophils, and bacteria are detected cytologically or by culture. Mixed populations of intracellular and extracellular bacteria are commonly seen. Gram staining may help to identify classes of organisms and direct initial antimicrobial therapy, because culture results take several days. Identification of gram-positive filamentous rods on cytology is most suggestive of *Actinomyces* spp or *Nocardia* spp (see Fig. 2), and it is important to note that these organisms, particularly *Actinomyces* spp, can be difficult to culture [27].

In human medicine, pleural fluid is further analyzed by measuring pH, lactate dehydrogenase (LDH) activity, and glucose concentration. The results of these tests help to categorize the severity of disease and to determine whether aggressive treatment options are indicated. If the pH of the fluid is less than 7.2, the fluid glucose concentration is less than 60 mg/dL, or the LDH activity is three times the upper limit of serum, aggressive therapy is warranted and the prognosis is guarded [29,30]. There is little information regarding the value of biochemical evaluation of pleural fluid in canine and feline pyothorax, however.

Other Diagnostic Imaging

Thoracic ultrasound may be indicated to help identify consolidated lung masses, mediastinal masses, and abscessed or neoplastic lung nodules. It also can be used to aid in sample procurement when only a small amount of pleural fluid is present and to determine the region of maximal effusion [26]. Advanced imaging is not commonly used in the diagnosis of pyothorax in veterinary medicine, although CT or MRI is often employed in human medicine to determine the extent of infection, to find pockets of fluid, or to identify an underlying cause.

TREATMENT

After diagnosis of pyothorax, there are several options for case management, none of which is known to be optimal. Table 1 compares the treatments and outcomes reported in studies of canine and feline pyothorax since the year 2000, and results vary widely. At a minimum, systemic antimicrobial therapy and supportive care are indicated. Thoracic drainage can be provided through needle thoracocentesis, thoracostomy tube placement, or thoracotomy. Although surgical intervention is aggressive, surgery is advantageous because it allows exploration of the thoracic cavity, identification and removal of an underlying cause, and thorough thoracic lavage. Thoracoscopy has been advocated as a less invasive alternative, although there are currently no veterinary studies that describe the use of this modality for pyothorax. Appropriate management of pleural empyema in human medicine is also controversial [31]. Most human patients are treated with antibiotics with or without repeat thoracocentesis, closed thoracostomy, or fibrinolytics [32]. Surgery is typically reserved for cases with complicated effusion or for cases refractory to conservative treatment.

Systemic Antimicrobial Therapy

Initial antimicrobial therapy should be broad spectrum to address the possible multiple organisms that could be involved. No single agent can be recommended to address all possible infective organisms; however, penicillins and penicillin derivatives are most commonly prescribed. Cefoxitin, enrofloxacin, and trimethoprim-sulfonamide have also been advocated as good empiric choices [11]. If clinical manifestations of sepsis are detected, it may be prudent to administer an antibiotic or combination of antibiotics that are effective against gram-positive and gram-negative aerobes and anaerobes. Once culture results are obtained, antimicrobial therapy should be directed at the identified organisms while maintaining efficacy against anaerobes, because these organisms can be difficult to isolate. *Actinomyces* spp infections are often suspected based on results of cytology rather than culture [27]. Long-term treatment (>6 weeks) with antibiotics in the β-lactam class is the treatment of choice for *Actinomyces* spp [21,27]. Other drugs that are commonly effective include clindamycin and chloramphenicol. *Nocardia* spp infections are not a common cause of pyothorax in dogs and cats; however, if they are diagnosed, long-term administration of sulfonamides may be indicated, and as with *Actinomyces* spp, treatment is prolonged [27].

Thoracocentesis

Needle aspiration of the pleural cavity can be diagnostic and therapeutic. After initial sampling of the fluid for diagnostic evaluation, removal of as much of the fluid as possible can provide considerable relief to severely affected animals. Because bilateral distribution of fluid is common, thoracocentesis should be performed on both sides of the thoracic cavity. Typically a 20- or 22-gauge needle is used, although butterfly catheters or small over-the-needle catheters are also used to perform thoracocentesis. The needle or catheter should be connected to extension tubing, which is connected to a three-way stopcock and large syringe. Thoracocentesis is best and most safely performed with the animal standing or in sternal recumbency. The needle is advanced into the pleural cavity at the level of the ventral third of the thorax and caudal to the fifth rib space to avoid iatrogenic injury to the heart. Retrieved fluid is evaluated cytologically and by aerobic and anaerobic culture. Repeat needle thoracocentesis is inefficient for complete thoracic drainage and is not recommended as a means of therapy because of the morbidity and risk associated with this technique. In human medicine, therapeutic needle thoracocentesis for purulent pleural

Table 1
Summary of recent retrospective pyothorax studies in dogs and cats

Authors	Geographic region	No. cases	Species	Treatment	Positive outcome in treated cases	Recurrence rate in cases with follow-up
Johnson and Martin [26]	United Kingdom	15	Canine	Single unilateral thoracic drainage in all cases[a]	100%	(0/15) 0%
Barrs et al [6]	Australia	27	Feline	6 (22%): died or euthanized without treatment; 18 (85%): thoracostomy tube; 2 (10%): antimicrobial therapy alone; 1 (5%): tube followed by surgery	78%	(2/14) 14%
Demetriou et al [10]	United Kingdom/Ireland	50	Canine and feline	10 (20%): surgery; 36 [72%]: thoracostomy tube drainage and lavage; 4 (8%): thoracostomy drainage alone	86%	(1/43) 2.3%
Mellanby et al [42]	United Kingdom	13	Canine	2 (15%): euthanized without treatment; 8 (62%): thoracostomy drainage alone; 3 (23%): surgery	64%	(0/7) 0%

Study	Country	Number	Species	Treatment	Survival	Mortality
Rooney and Monnet [11]	United States	26	Canine	7 (27%): thoracostomy drainage; 12 (46%): thoracostomy drainage followed by surgery; 7 (27%): surgery within 48 hours[b]	58%	(3/26) 11.6%
Waddell et al [13]	United States	80	Feline	21 (26%): euthanized without treatment; 5 (6%): thoracostomy drainage followed by surgery; 3 (4%): needle drainage; 48 (60%): thoracostomy tube; 3 (4%): antimicrobials alone[c]	66.10%	(1/17) 5.8%
Piek and Robben [25]	The Netherlands	9	Canine	9 (100%): systemic antibiotics with thoracostomy drainage and thoracic lavage[d]	100%	(0/8) 0%

[a]No dog had evidence of pulmonary masses, lung consolidation, or granular pleural effusion.
[b]Treatment was 5.4 times as likely to fail in dogs treated medically as in dogs treated surgically.
[c]Survival rate for the surgery group (5 of 5 dogs) was significantly (P = .024) higher compared with the nonsurgery group (34 [62.9%] of 54 dogs).
[d]All hunting dogs, but there was no evidence of migrating plant material.

effusion is considered an outdated modality [30]. If further drainage is indicated, thoracostomy tube placement is warranted.

Thoracostomy Tube

Needle aspiration of the pleural cavity is often ineffective for complete drainage of the pleural cavity, because fluid is typically thick and flocculated and tends to reaccumulate rapidly. Unilateral or bilateral thoracostomy tubes are placed to facilitate complete thoracic drainage. In dogs and cats, the right and left pleural cavities are widely believed to communicate through an imperforate mediastinum; therefore, septic pleural effusion is rarely isolated to a single hemithorax. The decision to place single or multiple tubes is based on the volume and distribution of fluid from thoracic radiographs. Sedation or general anesthesia is usually required for thoracostomy tube placement. Proper placement of a thoracostomy tube is through a skin incision in the dorsal third of the thoracic cavity at the level of the tenth to twelfth intercostal space. The tube is advanced through a generous subcutaneous tunnel in a caudodorsal-to-cranioventral direction and enters the pleural cavity through the midthoracic level of the seventh or eighth intercostal space. Once the tube is secured, placement should be verified on lateral and dorsoventral thoracic radiographs (Fig. 4). Pleural drainage may be intermittent or continuous. Continuous suction is labor- and equipment-intensive and is often not used for pyothorax because it has not been shown to be advantageous over intermittent drainage [6,33]. After tube placement and initial thoracic drainage, intermittent suction is typically performed every 2 to 6 hours for the first 24 to 48 hours. The volume and character of thoracic fluid should be closely monitored. Complications of thoracostomy tubes include kinking, clogging, inadvertent removal, and risk of ascending nosocomial infections.

Thoracic lavage is commonly performed in canine patients but is controversial in cats. Typically, warmed sterile isotonic solution at a rate of 10 to 20 mL/kg is instilled into the thoracic cavity after drainage. The fluid is left in place for 5 to 10 minutes, and the pleural cavity is then drained. Up to 75% of the instilled volume should be retrieved [34]. One recent study examining feline pyothorax concluded that thoracic lavage was not recommended [13]. Thoracic lavage was thought to be advantageous in a small case series of pyothorax in hunting dogs, however [25]. The risks of thoracic lavage include instillation of a large amount of fluid into a closed space, followed by an inability to retrieve it, as well as introduction of nosocomial infection if aseptic technique is not followed. There is also one report of a cat becoming hypokalemic when sterile saline at a rate of 50 mL/kg was used to lavage the thoracic cavity [6].

There is no known advantage to lavaging the thoracic cavity of dogs or cats with anything other than sterile physiologic solutions. In human medicine, the use of intrapleural fibrinolytic agents is common. Intrapleural injection of streptokinase was shown to facilitate pleural drainage when the fluid is thick and flocculated [35]. Urokinase and tissue plasminogen activator have also been

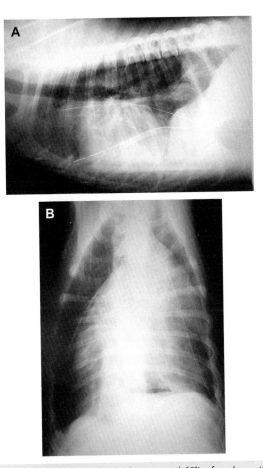

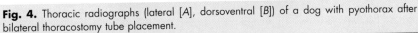

Fig. 4. Thoracic radiographs (lateral [A], dorsoventral [B]) of a dog with pyothorax after bilateral thoracostomy tube placement.

shown to be effective [36,37]. Recent data suggest that the use of fibrinolytic agents does not influence the outcome in human patients with pleural infection, however [38,39]. Some veterinary clinicians advocate addition of heparin to lavage fluid (1500 U per 100 mL), although there are no data to support the use of fibrinolytic agents in veterinary patients.

Criteria for determining failure of conservative management of pyothorax have not been determined, although most reports recommend that if there is no improvement in 48 to 72 hours or if there is clinical deterioration in the face of medical therapy, more aggressive methods of treatment are indicated. Recent studies have shown a benefit to surgical intervention. Surgical treatment was 5.4 times more likely to be successful in dogs than medical therapy, and cats that underwent surgery had a higher survival rate than those treated medically [11,13]. Excellent outcomes have been documented in dogs and cats with conservative management alone, however [6,26]. Recently, a study described 15 dogs that were managed with single unilateral thoracostomy tube drainage and long-term antimicrobial therapy [26]. All dogs had a complete recovery, and there was no evidence or recurrence.

Thoracotomy

Surgical exploration of the thoracic cavity is indicated if there is failure of medical therapy, a distinct underlying cause has been identified, mediastinal or pulmonary lesions are found on thoracic radiographs, or *Actinomyces* spp infection is suspected [11].

In human medicine, invasive procedures are found to be necessary when effusion is flocculated or consumes more than 50% of the hemithorax; when there is a positive Gram stain or culture; or when the purulent fluid has a pH less than 7.20, a glucose level less than 60, or an LDH level more than three times the upper limit of serum [30].

The most common surgical approach to the thorax is through a median sternotomy. This approach allows for complete exploration of the entire thoracic cavity. The objectives of surgery are to remove fluid and infected or necrotic tissue, debride pleural surfaces, identify and remove any foreign material, and lavage the entire pleural cavity to decrease the number of bacteria and allow better penetration of antimicrobials. Lung lobectomy or subtotal pericardiectomy may be indicated if these tissues are thickened or abscessed. Resected tissue should be submitted for additional culture and histopathologic examination. If not already placed, bilateral thoracostomy tubes are placed, and management continues similar to that described previously.

Thoracoscopy

Video-assisted thoracoscopic surgery (VATS) is a minimally invasive procedure that allows examination of the thoracic cavity. Although not yet described in veterinary medicine, VATS has been advocated as a method for treatment of septic pleural effusions in human medicine. It has been described to have a bridging role between conservative and aggressive management [30]. In a retrospective study in human medicine, VATS was found to be an effective definitive treatment for empyema, resulting in shorter hospital stays when compared with patients who underwent thoracostomy tube drainage alone, thoracostomy tube drainage with fibrinolytic administration, and thoracotomy [31]. Prospective randomized studies examining the role of VATS in septic pleural effusions are still needed, however [40]. The advantages of VATS are that it allows for exploration of the thoracic cavity, disruption of adhesions, complete drainage of the pleural cavity, and optimal thoracostomy tube placement [41].

PROGNOSIS

The prognosis for pyothorax is highly variable, and the argument of medical versus surgical therapy has yet to be decided (see Table 1). Mortality rates vary from 0% to 42%; however, animals are often euthanized without treatment because of poor prognosis, financial constraints, or the potential for recurrence [6,11,13,25,26]. Recurrence rates are also variable but are thought to be more of a concern for *Actinomyces* spp or *Nocardia* spp infections [11,27]. As veterinary medicine advances, thoracoscopy should be considered as another treatment modality for dogs and cats with pyothorax.

References

[1] Evans HE. The respiratory system. In: Evans HE, editor. Miller's anatomy of the dog. Philadelphia: WB Saunders; 1993. p. 463–93.

[2] Von Recum AF. The mediastinum and hemothorax, pyothorax, and pneumothorax in the dog. J Am Vet Med Assoc 1977;171(6):531–3.

[3] Rigby M, Zylak CJ, Wood LD. The effect of lobar atelectasis on pleural fluid distribution in dogs. Radiology 1980;136(3):603–7.

[4] Padrid P. Canine and feline pleural disease. Vet Clin North Am Small Anim Pract 2000;30(6):1295–307.

[5] Scott JA, Macintire DK. Canine pyothorax: pleural anatomy and pathophysiology. Compendium on Continuing Education for the Practicing Veterinarian 2003;25(3):172–9.

[6] Barrs VR, Allan GS, Martin P, et al. Feline pyothorax: a retrospective study of 27 cases in Australia. J Feline Med Surg 2005;7(4):211–22.

[7] Stork CK, Hamaide AJ, Schwedes C, et al. Hemiurothorax following diaphragmatic hernia and kidney prolapse in a cat. J Feline Med Surg 2003;5(2):91–6.

[8] Agostini E. Mechanics of the pleural space. Physiol Rev 1972;52(1):57–128.

[9] Black LF. The pleural space and pleural fluid. Mayo Clin Proc 1972;47(7):493–506.

[10] Dementriou JL, Foale RD, Ladlow J, et al. Canine and feline pyothorax; a retrospective study of 50 cases in the UK and Ireland. J Small Anim Pract 2002;43(9):388–94.

[11] Rooney MB, Monnet E. Medical and surgical treatment of pyothorax in dogs: 26 cases (1991–2001). J Am Vet Med Assoc 2002;221(1):86–92.

[12] Davies C, Forrester SD. Pleural effusion in cats: 82 cases (1987 to 1995). J Small Anim Pract 1996;37(5):217–24.

[13] Waddell LS, Brady CA, Drobatz KJ. Risk factors, prognostic indicators, and outcome of pyothorax in cats: 80 cases (1986–1999). J Am Vet Med Assoc 2002;221(6):819–24.

[14] Noone KE. Pleural effusions and diseases of the pleura. Vet Clin North Am Small Anim Pract 1995;15(5):1069–84.

[15] Brennan KE, Ihrke PJ. Grass awn migration in dogs and cats: a retrospective study of 182 cases. J Am Vet Med Assoc 1983;182(11):1201–4.

[16] Greene CE, Reinero CN. Bacterial respiratory infections. In: Greene CE, editor. Infectious diseases of the dog and cat. 3rd edition. St. Louis (MO): Elsevier; 2006. p. 866–82.

[17] Frendin J. Pyogranulomatous pleuritis with empyema in hunting dogs. Zentralbl Veterinarmed A 1997;44(3):167–78.

[18] Lotti U, Niebauer GW. Tracheobronchial foreign bodies of plant origin in 153 hunting dogs. Compendium on Continuing Education for the Practicing Veterinarian 1992;14(7):900–4.

[19] Buergelt CD. Pleural effusion in cats. Vet Med 2002;97(11):812–8.

[20] Jonas LD. Feline pyothorax: a retrospective study of twenty cases. J Am Anim Hosp Assoc 1983;19:865–71.

[21] Love DN, Jones RF, Bailey M, et al. Isolation and characterisation of bacteria from abscesses in the subcutis of cats. J Med Microbiol 1979;12(2):207–12.

[22] Gaskell RM, Radford AS, Dawson S, et al. Feline infectious respiratory disease. In: Chandler EA, Gaskell EA, Gaskell CJ, editors. Feline medicine and therapeutics. 3rd edition. Oxford (UK): Blackwell; 2004. p. 577–95.

[23] Walker AL, Jang SS, Hirsh DC. Bacteria associated with pyothorax of dogs and cats: 98 cases (1989–1998). J Am Vet Med Assoc 2000;216(3):359–63.

[24] Jang SS, Breher JE, Dabaco LA, et al. Organisms isolated from dogs and cats with anaerobic infections and susceptibility to selected antimicrobial agents. J Am Vet Med Assoc 1997;210(11):1610–4.

[25] Piek CJ, Robben JH. Pyothorax in nine dogs. Vet Q 2000;22(2):107–11.

[26] Johnson MS, Martin MWS. Successful medical treatment of 15 dogs with pyothorax. J Small Anim Pract 2007;48(1):12–6.

[27] Edwards DF. Actinomycosis and nocardiosis. In: Greene CE, editor. Infectious diseases of the dog and cat. 3rd edition. St. Louis (MO): Elsevier; 2006. p. 451–61.

[28] Robertson SA, Stoddart ME, Evans RJ, et al. Thoracic empyema in the dog: a report of twenty-two cases. J Small Anim Pract 1983;24(2):103–19.

[29] Light RW, MacGregor MI, Ball WC Jr, et al. Diagnostic significance of pleural fluid pH and PCO2. Chest 1973;64(5):591–6.

[30] Light RW. Parapneumonic effusions and empyema. Proc Am Thorac Soc 2006;3(1):75–80.

[31] Luh SP, Liu HP. Video-assisted thoracic surgery the past, present status and the future. J Zhejiang Univ Sci B 2006;7(2):118–28.

[32] Colice GL, Curtis A, Deslauriers J, et al. Medical and surgical treatment of parapneumonic effusions: an evidence-based guideline. Chest 2000;118(4):1158–71.

[33] Scott JA, Macintire DK. Canine pyothorax: clinical presentation, diagnosis, and treatment. Compendium on Continuing Education for the Practicing Veterinarian 2003;25(3): 180–94.

[34] Hawkins EC, Fossum TW. Medical and surgical management of pleural effusion. In: Bonagura JD, Kirk RW, editors. Kirk's current veterinary therapy: small animal practice XIII. Philadelphia: WB Saunders; 2000. p. 819–25.

[35] Tillett WS, Sherry S, Read CT. The use of streptokinase-streptodornase in the treatment of postpneumonic empyema. J Thorac Surg 1951;21(3):275–97.

[36] Bouros D, Schiza S, Patsourakis G, et al. Intrapleural streptokinase versus urokinase in the treatment of complicated parapneumonic effusions: a prospective, double-blind study. Am J Respir Crit Care Med 1997;11(1):265–8.

[37] Skeete DA, Rutherford EJ, Schlidt SA, et al. Intrapleural tissue plasminogen activator for complicated pleural effusions. J Trauma 2004;57(6):1178–83.

[38] Maskell NA, Davies CW, Nunn AJ, et al. First Multicenter Intrapleural Sepsis Trial (MIST1) group. U.K. controlled trial of intrapleural streptokinase for pleural infection. N Engl J Med 2005;352(9):865–74.

[39] Rahman NM, Chapman SJ, Davies RJ. The approach to the patient with a parapneumonic effusion. Clin Chest Med 2006;27(2):253–66.

[40] Gates RL, Caniano DA, Hayes JR, et al. Does VATS provide optimal treatment of empyema in children? A systematic review. J Pediatr Surg 2004;39(3):381–6.

[41] Silen ML, Naunheim KS. Thoracoscopic approach to the management of empyema thoracis: indications and results. Chest Surg Clin N Am 1996;6:491–9.

[42] Mellanby RJ, Villers E, Herrtage ME. Canine pleural and mediastinal effusion: a retrospective study of 81 cases. J Small Anim Pract 2002;43(10):447–51.

Nutritional Considerations for Animals with Pulmonary Disease

Scott J. Campbell, BVSc (Hons), MACVSc*

WALTHAM UCVMC-SD Clinical Nutrition Program, University of California Veterinary
Medical Center–San Diego, 10435 Sorrento Valley Road, Suite 101, San Diego, CA 92121, USA

Respiratory disease can result in malnutrition from anorexia secondary to severe dyspnea or development of a hypermetabolic state secondary to endocrine alterations and cytokine production [1,2]. Malnutrition from deficient nutrient intake may, in turn, adversely affect many factors clinically important to animals with pulmonary disease, including ventilatory drive in response to hypoxia, respiratory muscle mass and function, tissue synthesis or repair, immune competence and incidence of pneumonia, surfactant production, and drug metabolism [3–11]. Many hospitalized animals are likely to become malnourished without appropriate nutrition support, and if malnutrition occurs, it is likely to result in increased morbidity and mortality [12]. As well as having a supportive role, certain nutritional modifications may be used to modulate the underlying disease state. Provision of nutrition support incurs additional cost, however, and is not without potential detriment. Careful consideration of the individual animal and frequent reassessment are required to ensure that optimal nutrition support is maintained. This article focuses on the emerging nutritional therapies and strategies that may prove to be useful in managing small animals with pulmonary disease. Many potential avenues for future research in dogs and cats remain to be investigated.

ANIMAL SELECTION USING NUTRITIONAL ASSESSMENT

It is generally advised to attempt to stabilize the animal before considering nutrition support to minimize the risk of exacerbating existing fluid, electrolyte, and acid-base balance disturbances [2,13]. Even once the animal is deemed sufficiently stable to allow initiation of nutritional support, the clinical and metabolic response should be closely monitored to ensure that adverse sequelae do not go unrecognized. An initial nutritional assessment should be performed as soon as practical after presentation to enable the animal to be classified as malnourished, at risk of becoming malnourished, or well nourished. Nutritional assessment helps with the decision of when to initiate nutritional support

*Australian Veterinary Consulting, 95 Chermside Road, East Ipswich, Queensland 4305, Australia. E-mail address: ausvetcon@hotmail.com

0195-5616/07/$ – see front matter
doi:10.1016/j.cvsm.2007.05.010

and also gives direction on diet selection, feeding strategy selection, and monitoring guidelines [14]. The benefits and risks with refeeding, along with the overall prognosis, should be considered when formulating a nutritional strategy. Rather than using potential adverse effects as an excuse not to provide nutrition support, it should be the aim of informed veterinary clinicians to use the modality most likely to supply benefit without significant risk to the individual animal whenever possible. Some initial metabolic abnormalities may actually improve with provision of appropriate nutrition support. For example, preexisting moderate hypertriglyceridemia can resolve with nutrition support, presumably as a result of attenuated endogenous lipolysis with provision of exogenous caloric support. Additional details on performing a thorough nutritional assessment can be found in several recent articles on critical care nutrition [2,13,14]. As a minimum, the nutritional assessment should involve a subjective assessment of the animal's current nutritional status, including assignment of a body condition score and consideration of recent body weight changes, calculation of the current voluntary daily caloric intake using information from the diet history and comparison of this value with the calculated resting energy requirement (RER) for an average animal of that body weight, and consideration of the illness and expected period of anorexia [14]. Nutritional assessment of small animals is currently performed using multiple subjective parameters, because readily available, reliable, and inexpensive objective indicators remain elusive.

NUTRITIONAL GOALS FOR ANIMALS WITH PULMONARY DISEASE

Initial nutritional goals for animals with any critical illness, including those with respiratory disease, include provision of adequate calories to attenuate further breakdown of endogenous tissues (a controlled rate of weight loss can be initiated later if desired in obese animals) and provision of adequate protein to promote a positive nitrogen balance. Although weight stability serves as a surrogate marker for such factors as improved ventilatory drive, greater respiratory muscle strength, improved tissue synthesis or repair, and maintenance of immune competence, the response of these more clinically relevant parameters to nutritional intervention is currently quite difficult to assess in individual patients. Weight stability might also be difficult to assess in animals that have variable hydration status, however. Another important nutritional goal is the provision of a nutrient profile that minimizes the risk of metabolic refeeding complications, most notably hypophosphatemia, hypokalemia, hypomagnesemia, and hyperglycemia. Other considerations for animals with pulmonary disease are discussed in this article in the section on key nutritional factors.

NUTRITION PLAN FOR ANIMALS WITH PULMONARY DISEASE

Formulation of a nutrition plan requires consideration of the feeding method to be used and the type of diet to be provided. The selection of a feeding method is influenced by such factors as the current voluntary daily caloric intake, anticipated required duration of nutritional support, gastrointestinal function and risk of aspiration pneumonia with enteral feeding, anesthetic risk, coagulation status, available vascular access, fluid tolerance, cost, and type of diet desired [14]. The selection of the type of diet to be provided is influenced by the nutrient levels desired, clinician access to particular diets, type of intravenous access available, the type and size of feeding tube available, the animal's disease condition, cost, and the type of feeding method desired [14]. Because the feeding method and the type of diet affect one another, these two factors must be considered together. Other points to consider when formulating a nutrition plan include whether to use continuous rate or intermittent feeding (continuous rate feeding may be better tolerated by some patients), the rate of introduction of nutrition support (goal daily caloric requirements are generally only achieved after 3 or 4 days of incremental increases), whether consistency of the plan is needed to allow assessment of the animal's response, and whether any treats or supplements to the base diet are desired. Some of the therapies used in animals with respiratory disease may also necessitate modifications to the diet or the feeding method (eg, surgical therapy, ventilatory support).

Enteral nutrition is the preferred route of nutrition support whenever possible because it is more physiologically normal, it assists with maintenance of gastrointestinal mucosal barrier function, it supplies some nutrients directly to the enterocytes, it is less expensive, and it requires less specialized equipment and facilities to administer than parenteral nutrition [11]. Although pulmonary aspiration is a concern in all critically ill patients, the human literature suggests that the risk is insufficient to withhold enteral nutrition support in most cases [15]. There is also some information indicating that provision of parenteral nutrition may directly impair pulmonary macrophage function [16]. Several studies have now shown that early enteral feeding (within 3 days of illness) is associated with improved outcome in human critical care patients [11]. If nasoesophageal or esophagostomy tubes are placed to allow provision of enteral nutrition support to anorexic animals, caution must be exercised to ensure that the tubes or wrapping does not adversely affect patient respiration. If megaesophagus and related aspiration pneumonia are suspected, oral and esophageal feeding should be avoided and gastrostomy feeding techniques may be preferred. When enteral feeding is not possible, such as in anesthetized animals on artificial ventilatory support, in which gastrointestinal motility may be impaired [17], parenteral nutrition support can be initiated as a bridging modality until a transition back to enteral nutrition can be achieved [18,19]. In situations in which only partial enteral nutrition is possible, a combination approach using enteral and parenteral nutrition support concurrently can be used. Drugs, such as cyproheptadine and diazepam, can be tested in an attempt to stimulate appetite, but the potential side effects should be considered. In the experience of the author, drugs have generally proven ineffective in stimulating appetite sufficiently to ensure adequate voluntary daily caloric intake. All standard critical care nutrition feeding methods can be used in animals with pulmonary disease. Table 1 lists some of the commonly used commercially available diets suitable for critical care nutrition in dogs and cats.

KEY NUTRITIONAL FACTORS FOR ANIMALS WITH PULMONARY DISEASE
Energy
The calculated RER for the current hydrated body weight is often used as the initial estimated daily caloric requirement for critically ill animals. Although, historically, it was recommended to feed at higher caloric intakes (eg, using illness energy requirements, disease factors, or stress factors), more recent veterinary publications advocate feeding at the calculated RER (inclusive of calories from protein) initially, because this value approximates daily caloric requirements of critically ill animals determined using indirect calorimetry, is sufficient to attenuate significant weight loss in most animals, and is believed to reduce many of the other adverse effects of malnutrition [2,13,19]. The exponential formula used by many nutritionists to calculate RER (kcal/d) is $70 \cdot$ (body weight in kilograms)$^{0.75}$. To the author's knowledge, no studies have yet been performed looking at the energy requirements of dogs and cats with pulmonary disease specifically. Previous daily caloric intake (when weight is stable) is often used for dogs and cats that are not critically ill unless weight loss is desired. To determine the previous daily caloric intake accurately, a diet history with foods and amounts consumed (including all treats and supplements) must be obtained. The calculated maintenance energy requirement (MER) for the current body weight can be used if the previously daily caloric intake cannot be calculated from the available diet history (eg, because of ad lib or variable feeding). A full list of multipliers used to calculate the MER from the RER is available in veterinary nutrition texts [20]. The most commonly used MER multipliers are: $1.2 \cdot$ RER for a neutered cat, $1.4 \cdot$ RER for an intact cat, $1.6 \cdot$ RER for a neutered dog, and $1.8 \cdot$ RER for an intact dog. It should be remembered that individual daily energy requirements can vary markedly from the average values calculated using these formulas; thus, reassessment and adjustment are required if they are used. It is essential that adequate nutrient precursors for synthesis of enzyme cofactors involved in energy production be provided, along with the energy substrates. Among the most likely nutrients to be depleted in critically ill anorexic dogs and cats are the B vitamins, particularly thiamin; thus, care should be taken to ensure that these are supplied at levels greater than the known nutritional requirements [18].

PROTEIN, AMINO ACIDS, AND PRODUCTS OF AMINO ACID METABOLISM
Extended periods of protein malnutrition may result in many adverse effects relevant to animals with pulmonary disease, including reduced immune competence, respiratory muscle weakness, and inadequate tissue synthesis or repair [13]. Studies have shown that provision of adequate nutrition support can

Table 1
A selection of commercially available enteral diets formulated for critical care

Therapeutic diet	Protein (% ME)	Fat (% ME)	Carbohydrate (% ME)	Kilocalories
Hill's Prescription Diet Canine/ Feline a/d canned[a]	33.2	55.2	11.6	180 per can
Royal Canin Veterinary Diet Canine Modified Formula canned[b]	12.9	46.5	40.6	619 per can
Royal Canin Veterinary Diet Canine Modified Formula dry[b]	12.4	32.5	55.1	367 per cup
Royal Canin Veterinary Diet Feline Modified Formula canned[b]	22.8	69.1	8.1	258 or 596 per can
Royal Canin Veterinary Diet Feline Modified Formula dry[b]	22.1	42.4	35.5	432 per cup
Purina Veterinary Diets Canine CV Cardiovascular canned[c]	12.3	53.4	34.3	638 per can
Purina Veterinary Diets Feline CV Cardiovascular canned[c]	32.6	49.8	17.6	223 per can
Purina Veterinary Diets Feline DM Diabetes Management canned[c]	49.0	44.0	7.0	194 per can
Purina Veterinary Diets Feline DM Diabetes Management dry[c]	51.7	37.0	11.3	592 per cup
Eukanuba Veterinary Diets Canine/Feline Maximum-Calorie canned[d]	29.0	66.0	5.0	340 per can
Eukanuba Veterinary Diets Canine Maximum-Calorie dry[d]	31.0	54.0	15.0	634 per cup
Eukanuba Veterinary Diets Feline Maximum-Calorie dry[d]	31.0	54.0	15.0	602 per cup
Abbott Animal Health Canine/ Feline Clinicare liquid[e]	30.0	45.0	25.0	1 kcal/mL
Abbott Animal Health Feline Clinicare RF liquid[e]	22.0	57.0	21.0	1 kcal/mL
Ross Human Vital HN powder (reconstituted to liquid)[e,f]	16.7	9.5	73.8	1 kcal/mL
Abbott Laboratories Human Pulmocare liquid[e,f]	16.7	55.1	28.2	1.5 kcal/mL

Current as of September 1, 2006.
[a]Hill's Pet Nutrition, Inc., Topeka, Kansas.
[b]Royal Canin USA, Inc., St. Charles, Missouri.
[c]Société des Produits Nestlé S.A., Vevey, Switzerland.
[d]The Iams Company, Dayton, Ohio.
[e]Abbott Laboratories, Abbott Park, Illinois.
[f]Human diets are not complete and balanced for long-term feeding to dogs and cats without appropriate supplementation.

improve nitrogen balance [21,22]. Dietary protein should be adequate to minimize catabolism and maintain metabolic protein demands. Most authors recommend that protein be provided to critically ill dogs and cats at a rate of 3 to 8 g per 100 kcal depending on species and disease state [2,13], a level that supplies approximately 10% to 32% of the total metabolizable energy (ME) as protein. Dogs and cats that have only pulmonary disease, without concurrent azotemia or hepatic encephalopathy, may safely be fed diets with protein contents at the higher end of this range, thus reducing the dependence on fat or carbohydrate to provide calories. Other authors have suggested that critically ill dogs should receive 25% to 45% of their total ME as protein and that critically ill cats should receive 30% to 50% of their total ME as protein unless the individual has uremia, hepatic encephalopathy, or excessive protein losses [12].

In addition to the total protein content of the diet, some individual amino acids and products of amino acid metabolism are worthy of specific consideration. All canine and feline enteral diets contain arginine, an essential amino acid that has been shown to improve nitrogen balance and immune function [13]. Supplementation of additional arginine greater than the known nutritional requirement to dogs and cats with pulmonary disease is of questionable benefit at this stage. Glutamine, a conditionally essential amino acid for dogs and cats, may be of benefit during periods of stress, but its expense and relative instability currently limit its use in veterinary patients [13]. The branched chain amino acids leucine, isoleucine, and valine can be metabolized directly in muscle tissue rather than in the liver and may supply an additional source of energy as well as having regulatory actions [12]. Research into the clinical utility of supplementing branched chain amino acids to critically ill animals is deficient at this time. L-carnitine, usually synthesized endogenously from lysine and methionine, is required for transport of long-chain fatty acids across the mitochondrial membrane for subsequent β-oxidation. Whether providing additional L-carnitine to animals with pulmonary disease already consuming diets with adequate levels of total protein, lysine, and methionine is of any benefit remains to be determined.

Electrolytes

Refeeding of previously anorexic patients, particularly with diets high in rapidly absorbed and metabolized carbohydrates, can result in hypophosphatemia, hypokalemia, and hypomagnesemia as part of the refeeding syndrome [18, 23–27]. These electrolyte alterations occur secondary to preexisting whole-body electrolyte depletion and intracellular movement with glucose uptake and glycolysis [18]. Refeeding syndrome can occur with parenteral, enteral, or oral feeding [18]. Hypophosphatemia is believed to result in clinical signs, including muscle weakness and respiratory insufficiency in human beings [25,26]. Hypokalemia and hypomagnesemia can also be associated with generalized muscle weakness that could exacerbate preexisting respiratory muscle dysfunction [26,28–32]. Sodium retention can occur as part of the refeeding syndrome and may exacerbate pulmonary edema if present [18]. As such, it is prudent to correct electrolyte abnormalities routinely before feeding and to monitor for electrolyte shifts with refeeding in all animals that may have experienced whole-body electrolyte depletion from extended periods of anorexia or prolonged ingestion of unbalanced diets. A recent human study indicated that instituting a routine electrolyte replacement protocol when refeeding patients requiring nutrition support alleviated the clinical consequences of refeeding syndrome [33].

Carbohydrate

Nutritional hypercapnia is an important complication recognized in human patients who have respiratory disease [9,34–37]. Initiation of routine nutritional support in human patients has been shown to increase endogenous carbon dioxide production, which can, in turn, necessitate introduction of or adjustments to such therapies as artificial ventilation [38,39]. Alteration of the nutrient profile of the diet can affect the respiratory quotient (RQ; ratio of moles of carbon dioxide produced to moles of oxygen consumed) that results from metabolism of energy substrates in the diet. The RQ that results from carbohydrate metabolism is 1.0, indicating that similar amounts of carbon dioxide are produced as oxygen is consumed. The RQ that results from metabolism of an average animal fat is 0.7, and the RQ that results from metabolism of an average meat protein is 0.8, indicating that less carbon dioxide is produced per unit of oxygen consumed [18]. When consideration is given to the actual volume of carbon dioxide produced per unit of energy generated, however, the numbers are different. Carbohydrate and protein are relatively equivalent, at approximately 200 L and 209 L of carbon dioxide produced per 1000 kcal, respectively, whereas the amount of carbon dioxide produced per unit of energy generated when fat is metabolized is markedly lower at approximately 155 L per 1000 kcal (assuming that the carbon dioxide behaves as an ideal gas and no energy storage occurs) [40]. Because of this, the level of carbohydrate is often restricted and the level of fat is increased as the source of nonprotein calories in the diet of people who have respiratory disease. A controlled study of human patients receiving assisted ventilation showed that feeding a low-carbohydrate diet rather than a standard diet resulted in reduction of $Paco_2$ and earlier weaning from the ventilator [34]. Provision of caloric intake beyond the animal's actual daily energy requirement may also result in undesirable alterations in the RQ, particularly if high-carbohydrate diets are used, because of increased carbon dioxide production with endogenous fat synthesis [11,13,41–47]. To the author's knowledge, studies reporting expired gas analysis of dogs and cats with pulmonary disease fed variable diet compositions and caloric loads have yet to be reported. A recent human study indicated that the RQ determined by indirect calorimetry could be used as a marker of respiratory tolerance to the nutrition support regimen, but the low sensitivity and specificity in detecting underfeeding or overfeeding of this analysis limit its use in fine-tuning the regimen [44].

Pulmocare (Abbott Laboratories, Abbott Park, Illinois) is an example of a human enteral product formulated specifically for patients who have respiratory disease. This product has a high calorie density (1.5 kcal/mL); low carbohydrate content for a human diet (28.2% carbohydrate on a ME basis); and added antioxidants, including vitamin C, vitamin E, and β-carotene. It should be noted that although the level of carbohydrates in this product would be considered restricted for people and dogs, it would not be considered restricted for cats, because many available feline diets contain 20% to 40% carbohydrate on a ME basis. It should also be remembered that human enteral products usually do not meet the full nutritional requirements of dogs and cats; as such, they are not suitable for extended feeding periods unless supplemented appropriately. Restriction of the carbohydrate content of the diet may also reduce the risk of the animal experiencing extended periods of hyperglycemia. This is desirable, because unmanaged hyperglycemia may result in reduced immune competence and has been shown to increase mortality in human intensive care patients [18,48–52].

Fat and Fatty Acids

Consumption of high-fat diets (>40% fat on a ME basis) may have additional benefits beyond reduction in the carbohydrate load, with such factors as higher energy density (kcal per unit of weight) and palatability also important for many critically ill animals [12]. Animals rapidly deplete body glycogen stores and are reliant on protein and fat metabolism for energy after a few days of anorexia. Because some dogs and cats may exhibit fat intolerance when fed high-fat diets, however, they must be monitored for diarrhea, pancreatitis, lipemia, or hypertriglyceridemia. Consideration should be given to the lipids and calories administered concurrently in fat-containing medications, such as a propofol infusion [18]. In addition, hypertriglyceridemia can result from carbohydrate overfeeding in patients receiving parenteral nutrition [18].

It may be possible to improve lung function by providing specific fatty acids that attenuate lung inflammation. Certain polyunsaturated fatty acids (PUFAs), such as Ω-3 PUFA eicosapentaenoic acid (EPA) and Ω-6 PUFA gamma-linolenic acid (GLA), have shown promise as immunomodulatory supplements in many species and disease conditions, including people who have acute respiratory distress syndrome [53]. Recent studies have shown that administration of an enteral nutrition formula supplemented with EPA, GLA, and antioxidants reduced pulmonary inflammation, improved gas exchange and tissue oxygenation, reduced the requirement for artificial ventilatory support, reduced the time spent in the intensive care unit, and reduced the frequency of development of new organ failure [53–56]. These changes are possibly attributable to anti-inflammatory, vasodilatory, or antioxidant effects. In contrast, a recent review of the effects of Ω-3 PUFA supplementation in people who have asthma found few significant beneficial effects [57]. Incorporation of medium-chain triglycerides into the lipid solution may also be of value for patients who have pulmonary disease receiving parenteral nutrition [18,58]; however, additional studies are needed to evaluate further whether any significant clinical effects can be obtained with this modification.

Antioxidants

The antioxidant content of the diet may also require consideration in animals with pulmonary disease. The lungs are continually exposed to relatively high oxygen concentrations and can also be subjected to a variety of environmental pollutants and irritants that generate reactive oxygen species, resulting in increased vulnerability to oxidant attack [59]. Inflammatory cells activated in the lung with infection or inflammation may also generate free radicals and oxidant injury [60]. Therapies used for respiratory conditions, such as oxygen therapy, chemotherapy, and radiation therapy, can also result in endogenous free radical generation. It has been shown that oxidized lipids in the diet of growing dogs may affect some measured parameters of antioxidant status and immune function [61]. A variety of antioxidant protective mechanisms are present in the lung but vary markedly among individuals [59]. There is increasing evidence in people that consumption of foods high in antioxidant vitamins may impart a protective effect on lung function [54–56,59,62–70]. The mechanism of this protective effect is speculated to involve maintenance of adequate antioxidant nutrient concentrations within the lung to prevent oxidant damage [54,59]. It is also possible that initial oxidative stress may initiate subsequent increases in the antioxidant protective mechanisms maintained by an individual [71].

The ideal combination and concentration of antioxidant nutrients in the diet of dogs and cats with various pulmonary conditions have yet to be determined, but a recent study in obese cats has shown that administration of a D-α-tocopherol–supplemented parenteral solution resulted in a higher concentration of red blood cell glutathione than in control cats given standard parenteral solutions [72]. It should not be forgotten that reactive oxygen species can be important for destroying microorganisms and intracellular signaling; thus, excessive suppression of their generation is not desirable [73]. Excessive supplementation of particular antioxidants may result in direct cell signaling effects or pro-oxidant effects and should be avoided until the clinical consequences of these additional effects are further understood [74,75].

PREBIOTIC AND PROBIOTIC CONTENT

Some authors are now speculating that lifelong or intermittent supplementation of diets with prebiotics or probiotics, already recognized to stimulate enterocyte and colonocyte proliferation, may support the development of normal immunologic mucosal tolerance, thus reducing the risk of allergic airway disease [76]. The clinical relevance of this modification in dogs and cats with pulmonary disease remains to be determined.

OTHER NUTRIENTS

All other nutrients should be supplied at levels sufficient to meet the known minimum requirements. Long-term administration of diets deficient in any nutrients known to be essential to dogs and cats is eventually likely to contribute to morbidity and mortality. For example, zinc deficiency may affect protein metabolism, resulting in impaired tissue synthesis or repair and reduced immune competence [12]. Copper and vitamin A deficiencies have also been reported to affect lung parenchymal tissue adversely [11]. Taurine deficiency may allow terminal activation and release of cytotoxic mediators from lung macrophages in cats [77]. Therefore, it is desirable to feed a diet known to be complete and balanced for the species being treated. If animals are fed at daily caloric intakes lower than their calculated RER for extended periods, consideration should be given to provision of a diet with higher concentrations of the key nutrients or supplementation of these nutrients in addition to the reduced dietary intake.

WEIGHT MANAGEMENT

Weight management is an important long-term consideration in overweight or obese animals with pulmonary disease. Obesity is one of the most common forms of malnutrition in dogs and cats and can be evaluated clinically by using body condition scoring or morphometric measurements [78]. Obesity has been established to have negative effects on the health and longevity of some breeds of dogs and may be associated with cardiorespiratory disease in individual animals [79–84]. Smaller and lighter breeds of dogs generally live longer than larger and heavier breeds; thus, whether the effect of obesity on longevity is present across all dog breeds remains to be determined. Obesity was also one of the factors associated with mortality in dogs with heat stoke in a recent study [85]. Some authors have also indicated that obesity may alter drug metabolism, requiring alterations in medication dosages to achieve therapeutic levels [86,87]. Whole-body plethysmography in dogs has demonstrated that obesity increases respiration rate, increases minute volume, reduces respiratory tidal volume, reduces inspiratory time, and reduces expiratory time [88,89]. Preliminary studies suggest that obesity increases airway reactivity to histamine and impairs the positive ventilatory response to doxapram hydrochloride [88,89]. There is increasing literature to indicate that adipose tissue produces several endocrine factors that may have proinflammatory properties [90]. Therefore, there are several possible reasons why obesity management can be beneficial for animals with pulmonary disease. Obesity-hypoventilation syndrome (Pickwickian syndrome) in human beings is characterized by chronic alveolar hypoventilation (often without hypercapnia) because of increased respiration workload, dysfunction of the respiratory centers, and repeated episodes of sleep apnea [91–93]. This condition is reversible with weight loss in people, and although the syndrome has not been described specifically in veterinary medicine, it is likely relevant to small animal patients.

An effective weight loss plan should encompass an initial animal evaluation and client education process, selection of an appropriate diet and feeding strategy, implementation of an appropriate exercise program, and regular reassessment with adjustments as needed to ensure an adequate rate of weight loss until the animal can be transitioned back to a maintenance diet. Canine and feline obesity was discussed in detail in a recent edition of this journal [90]. For reader convenience, tables of the commercially available canine and feline diets suitable for active weight loss are provided with this article (Tables 2 and 3). Pet food manufacturers often make adjustments to their diets over time; thus, it would be appropriate to recheck the information contained within these

Table 2
Commercially available canine diets formulated for active weight loss

Therapeutic diet	Protein (% ME)	Fat (% ME)	Carbohydrate (% ME)	Fiber (g/1000 kcal)	Moisture (% as fed)	Density (g per can or cup)	Kilocalories
Hill's Prescription Diet Canine r/d canned[a]	29.7	24.6	45.7	71	78	404	296 kcal per 14.25-oz can
Hill's Prescription Diet Canine r/d dry[a]	29.8	24.9	45.3	78	11	82	220 kcal/cup
Purina OM Canine Formula canned[b]	51.2	23.6	25.2	77.7	82	354	189 kcal per 12.5-oz can
Purina OM Canine Formula dry[b]	34.9	17.7	47.4	34.6	12	101	276 kcal/cup
Royal Canin Canine CC HP canned[c]	42.6	53.1	4.3	6.3	84.8	360	263 kcal per 12.7-oz can
Royal Canin Canine CC 32 HP dry[c]	37.6	23.5	38.9	8.5	8.5	66	234 kcal/cup
Royal Canin Canine CC HF canned[c]	25.3	29.6	45.1	24.5	75.6	360	346 kcal per 12.7-oz can
Royal Canin Canine CC 26 HF dry[c]	34.4	28.1	37.5	56	8.5	81	232 kcal/cup
Eukanuba Canine Restricted Calorie canned[d]	31	39	30	5.4	78	397	445 kcal per 14-oz can
Eukanuba Canine Restricted Calorie dry[d]	24	17	59	5.1	10	65	238 kcal/cup
Pedigree Canine Weight Loss dry[e]	53	21	26	8.9	12	73	246 kcal/cup

Current as of September 1, 2006.
[a]Hill's Pet Nutrition, Inc., Topeka, Kansas.
[b]Société des Produits Nestlé S.A., Vevey, Switzerland.
[c]Royal Canin USA, Inc., St. Charles, Missouri.
[d]The Iams Company, Dayton, Ohio.
[e]Mars, Incorporated, Hackettstown, New Jersey.

Table 3
Commercially available feline diets formulated for active weight loss

Therapeutic diet	Protein (% ME)	Fat (% ME)	Carbohydrate (% ME)	Fiber (g/1000 kcal)	Moisture (% as fed)	Density (g per can or cup)	Kilocalories
Hill's Prescription Diet Feline r/d canned[a]	38.2	25.2	36.6	55	78	156	116 kcal per 5.5-oz can
Hill's Prescription Diet Feline r/d L&C canned[a]	41.3	24.5	34.2	50	78	156	114 kcal per 5.5-oz can
Hill's Prescription Diet Feline r/d dry[a]	40.4	24.9	34.7	41	11	88	263 kcal/cup
Hill's Prescription Diet Feline m/d canned[a]	45.7	40.7	13.6	15	78	156	156 kcal per 5.5-oz can
Hill's Prescription Diet Feline m/d dry	43.0	44.1	12.9	13	10	122	480 kcal/cup
Purina OM Feline Formula canned[b]	43.1	34.4	22.5	26	77	156	150 kcal per 5.5-oz can
Purina OM Feline Formula dry[b]	56.2	20.5	23.3	17.6	11	105	340 kcal/cup
Royal Canin Feline CC HP canned[c]	45.4	46.5	8.1	5.1	83.4	165	130 kcal per 5.8-oz can
Royal Canin Feline CC HP pouch[c]	43.9	36	20.1	7.7	82.3	85	66 kcal per 3-oz pouch
Royal Canin Feline CC 38 HP dry[c]	44.4	23.4	32.2	11.2	7	68	235 kcal/cup
Royal Canin Feline CC HF canned	28.4	44	27.6	18.7	76.6	170	164 kcal per 6-oz can
Royal Canin Feline CC 29 HF dry[c]	36.1	26.7	37.2	43	7	83	251 kcal/cup
Eukanuba Feline Restricted Calorie canned[d]	40	41	19	2.1	87	170	204 kcal per 6-oz can
Eukanuba Feline Restricted Calorie dry[d]	34	23	43	5.4	8.5	78	277 kcal/cup

Current as of September 1, 2006.

[a]Hill's Pet Nutrition, Inc., Topeka, Kansas.

[b]Société des Produits Nestlé S.A., Vevey, Switzerland.

[c]Royal Canin USA, Inc., St. Charles, Missouri.

[d]The Iams Company, Dayton, Ohio.

tables to ensure that it is still accurate before use. Dogs and cats can be started at a total daily caloric intake equivalent to 80% of their previous daily caloric intake when weight is stable. If the previous daily caloric intake cannot be calculated from the diet history because of ad lib or variable feeding, dogs can be started at a total daily caloric intake equivalent to the calculated RER using the formula RER (kcal/d) $= 70 \cdot$ (body weight in kilograms)$^{0.75}$, and cats can be started at a total daily caloric intake equivalent to 80% of the calculated RER using the same formula. Up to 10% of total daily calories can be provided as unbalanced treats (commercial pet treats and human foods) without risk of unbalancing the base diet. As well as reducing the total daily caloric intake, an increase in the daily energy expenditure is usually advised for animals that are able to tolerate exercise. Regardless of the initial total daily caloric intake suggested, it is critical to recheck the rate of weight loss regularly to ensure that an appropriate rate is achieved. A rate of weight loss from 0.5% to 2% of current body weight per week is considered reasonable, with slower rates suggested for animals that may be metabolically unstable. Once the desired clinical response and body condition score have been achieved, the animal may be transitioned to a low-calorie/light/lite maintenance diet designed to assist with preventing recurrent weight gain.

GASTROINTESTINAL DISEASE MANAGEMENT

Diet can also be considered a potential source of allergens or irritants manifesting as respiratory disease [94]. Recently published studies have suggested a relation between respiratory disease and gastrointestinal disease (diagnosed by endoscopy and histopathologic examination) in brachycephalic dogs [95,96]. Possible contributors to this relation suggested by the authors include pharyngeal inflammation secondary to the gastrointestinal disease or gastroesophageal reflux secondary to the respiratory disease. The detection and treatment of concurrent gastrointestinal disease have been proposed to improve the results of upper airway surgery in brachycephalic dogs with respiratory disease [95], although a study with a suitable control group would be needed to prove benefit. Although the exact mechanism behind this relation remains to be conclusively determined, the potential benefit justifies assessment for the concurrent presence of gastrointestinal disease in animals with respiratory disease, and appropriate management (dietary and medical) should be instituted.

MONITORING AND REASSESSMENT

Regular monitoring for metabolic, mechanical, and septic complications is essential to ensure that modifications are made to the nutrition plan over time to provide maximal benefit and minimal risk to the individual animal. It is also important to record the current nutrition plan and any complications in the animal's medical record, such that this information is available when making alterations to the nutrition plan. Along with the amount of food offered, it is important to record the actual amount consumed and any regurgitation or vomiting that occurs.

SUMMARY

Many dogs and cats with pulmonary disease benefit from timely nutritional assessment and provision of appropriate nutrition support. The exact nature of the support required varies depending on the severity and type of pulmonary disease. Obese animals with chronic respiratory disease may benefit from weight loss, whereas animals with acute pulmonary disease may experience malnutrition and require aggressive nutrition support interventions. Standard critical care feeding methods can be used in animals with pulmonary disease, but selection or formulation of a diet with specific modifications may reduce morbidity and mortality. Key nutritional factors to consider include energy, protein, fat, carbohydrate, specific amino acids, specific fatty acids, electrolytes, antioxidants, prebiotic and probiotic content, weight management, and gastrointestinal disease management. Regular monitoring and reassessment of the nutrition plan is needed to ensure that the animal obtains optimal support. Many avenues remain to be investigated in the field of nutrition for animals with pulmonary disease; thus, additional data to assist with selection of the feeding method and the diet are likely to become available in the future.

References

[1] Cerra FB, Benitez MR, Blackburn GL, et al. Applied nutrition in ICU patients: a consensus statement of the American College of Chest Physicians. Chest 1997;111(3):769–78.

[2] Chan DL. Nutritional support of critically ill patients. WALTHAM Focus 2006;16(3):9–15.

[3] Burkholder WJ, Swecker WS. Nutritional influences on immunity. Semin Vet Med Surg (Small Anim) 1990;5:154–66.

[4] Chan DL. Parenteral nutrition support. In: Ettinger SJ, Feldman EC, editors. Textbook of veterinary internal medicine. St Louis (MI): Elsevier Saunders; 2005. p. 586–91.

[5] Crane SW. Nutritional aspects of wound healing. Semin Vet Med Surg (Small Anim) 1989;4:263–7.

[6] Fettman MJ, Phillips RW. Dietary effects on drug metabolism. In: Hand MS, Thatcher CD, Remillard RL, et al, editors. Small animal clinical nutrition. 4th edition. Topeka (KS): Mark Morris Institute; 2000. p. 923–39.

[7] Hart N, Tounian P, Clement A, et al. Nutritional status as an important predictor of diaphragm strength in young patients with cystic fibrosis. Am J Clin Nutr 2004;80(5): 1201–6.

[8] Mowatt-Larssen CA, Brown RO. Specialized nutritional support in respiratory disease. Clin Pharm 1993;12(4):276–92.

[9] Pingleton SK. Nutrition in chronic critical illness. Clin Chest Med 2001;22(1):149–63.

[10] Remillard RL, Thatcher CD. Parenteral nutritional support in the small animal patient. Vet Clin North Am Small Anim Pract 1989;19:1287–306.

[11] Sherman MS. Parenteral nutrition and cardiopulmonary disease. In: Rombeau JL, Rolandelli RH, editors. Clinical nutrition parenteral nutrition. 3rd edition. Philadelphia: W.B. Saunders Company; 2001. p. 335–52.

[12] Elliott DA, Biourge V. Critical care nutrition. WALTHAM Focus 2006;16(3):30–4.

[13] Remillard RL. Nutritional support in critical care patients. Vet Clin North Am Small Anim Pract 2002;32(5):1145–64.

[14] Michel KE. Deciding who needs nutritional support. WALTHAM Focus 2006;16(3): 16–20.

[15] Mullan H, Roubenoff RA, Roubenoff R. Risk of pulmonary aspiration among patients receiving enteral nutrition support. JPEN J Parenter Enteral Nutr 1992;16(2):160–4.

[16] Shou J, Lappin J, Daly JM. Impairment of pulmonary macrophage function with total parenteral nutrition. Ann Surg 1994;219:291–7.

[17] Lee TL, Ang SB, Dambisya YM, et al. The effect of propofol on human gastric and colonic muscle contractions. Anesth Analg 1999;89(5):1246–9.

[18] Btaiche IF, Khalidi N. Metabolic complications of parenteral nutrition in adults, part 1. Am J Health Syst Pharm 2004;61:1938–49.

[19] Campbell SJ, Karriker MJ, Fascetti AJ. Central and peripheral parenteral nutrition. WALTHAM Focus 2006;16(3):21–9.

[20] Thatcher CD, Hand MS, Remillard RL. Small animal clinical nutrition: an iterative process. In: Hand MS, Thatcher CD, Remillard RL, et al, editors. Small animal clinical nutrition. 4th edition. Topeka (KS): Mark Morris Institute; 2000. p. 1–19.

[21] Chandler ML, Guilford WG, Maxwell A, et al. A pilot study of protein sparing in healthy dogs using peripheral parenteral nutrition. Res Vet Sci 2000;69:47–52.

[22] Mauldin GE, Reynolds AJ, Mauldin GN, et al. Nitrogen balance in clinically normal dogs receiving parenteral nutrition solutions. Am J Vet Res 2001;62:912–20.

[23] Brooks MJ, Melnik G. The refeeding syndrome: an approach to understanding its complications and preventing its occurrence. Pharmacotherapy 1995;15:713–26.

[24] Crook MA, Hally V, Panteli JV. The importance of the refeeding syndrome. Nutrition 2001;17(7–8):632–7.

[25] Kraft MD, Btaiche IF, Sacks GS. Review of the refeeding syndrome. Nutr Clin Pract 2005;20(6):625–33.

[26] Marinella MA. Refeeding syndrome and hypophosphatemia. J Intensive Care Med 2005;20(3):155–9.

[27] Solomon SM, Kirby DF. The refeeding syndrome: a review. JPEN J Parenter Enteral Nutr 1990;14:90–7.

[28] Dhingra S, Solven F, Wilson A, et al. Hypomagnesemia and respiratory muscle power. Am Rev Respir Dis 1984;129(3):497–8.

[29] Landon RA, Young EA. Role of magnesium in regulation of lung function. J Am Diet Assoc 1993;93(6):674–7.

[30] Phillips SL, Polzin DJ. Clinical disorders of potassium homeostasis. Hyperkalemia and hypokalemia. Vet Clin North Am Small Anim Pract 1998;28(3):545–64.

[31] Rochester DF, Arora NS. Respiratory muscle failure. Med Clin North Am 1983;67(3): 573–97.

[32] Tong GM, Rude RK. Magnesium deficiency in critical illness. J Intensive Care Med 2005;20(1):3–17.

[33] Flesher ME, Archer KA, Leslie BD, et al. Assessing the metabolic and clinical consequences of early enteral feeding in the malnourished patient. JPEN J Parenter Enteral Nutr 2005;29(2):108–17.

[34] al-Saady NM, Blackmore CM, Bennett ED. High fat, low carbohydrate, enteral feeding lowers $PaCO_2$ and reduces the period of ventilation in artificially ventilated patients. Intensive Care Med 1989;15(5):290–5.

[35] Angelillo VA, Bedi S, Durfee D, et al. Effects of low and high carbohydrate feedings in ambulatory patients with chronic obstructive pulmonary disease and chronic hypercapnia. Ann Intern Med 1985;103(6):883–5.

[36] Bartlett RH, Dechert RE, Mault JR, et al. Metabolic studies in chest trauma. J Thorac Cardiovasc Surg 1984;87(4):503–8.

[37] Cai B, Zhu Y, Ma Y, et al. Effect of supplementing a high-fat, low-carbohydrate enteral formula in COPD patients. Nutrition 2003;19(3):229–32.

[38] Covelli HD, Black JW, Olsen MS, et al. Respiratory failure precipitated by high carbohydrate loads. Ann Intern Med 1981;95(5):579–81.

[39] Trunet P, Dreyfuss D, Bonnet JL, et al. Increase in partial arterial carbon dioxide pressure due to enteral nutrition during artificial ventilation. Presse Med 1983;12(46):2927–30.

[40] Baldwin RL. Animal energetic models: historical development of bases for feeding system models. In: Baldwin RL, editor. Modeling ruminant digestion and metabolism. London: Chapman & Hall; 1995. p. 118–47.

[41] Guenst JM, Nelson LD. Predictors of total parenteral nutrition-induced lipogenesis. Chest 1994;105(2):553–9.

[42] Kiiski R, Takala J. Hypermetabolism and efficiency of CO_2 removal in acute respiratory failure. Chest 1994;105(4):1198–203.

[43] Liposky JM, Nelson LD. Ventilatory response to high caloric loads in critically ill patients. Crit Care Med 1994;22(5):796–802.

[44] McClave SA, Lowen CC, Kleber MJ, et al. Clinical use of the respiratory quotient obtained from indirect calorimetry. JPEN J Parenter Enteral Nutr 2003;27(1):21–6.

[45] Schwarz JM, Chiolero R, Revelly JP, et al. Effects of enteral carbohydrates on de novo lipogenesis in critically ill patients. Am J Clin Nutr 2000;72(4):940–5.

[46] Tappy L, Schwarz JM, Schneiter P, et al. Effects of isoenergetic glucose-based or lipid-based parenteral nutrition on glucose metabolism, de novo lipogenesis, and respiratory gas exchanges in critically ill patients. Crit Care Med 1998;26(5):860–7.

[47] Van Den Berg B, Stam H. Metabolic and respiratory effects of enteral nutrition in patients during mechanical ventilation. Intensive Care Med 1988;14(3):206–11.

[48] Digman C, Borto D, Nasraway SA Jr. Hyperglycemia in the critically ill. Nutr Clin Care 2005;8(2):93–101.

[49] Gearhart MM, Parbhoo SK. Hyperglycemia in the critically ill patient. AACN Clin Issues 2006;17(1):50–5.

[50] McMahon MM. Management of parenteral nutrition in acutely ill patients with hyperglycemia. Nutr Clin Pract 2004;19(2):120–8.

[51] Turina M, Fry DE, Polk HC Jr. Acute hyperglycemia and the innate immune system: clinical, cellular, and molecular aspects. Crit Care Med 2005;33(7):1624–33.

[52] Van Den Berghe G, Wouters PJ, Weekers F, et al. Intensive insulin therapy in critically ill patients. N Engl J Med 2001;345:1359–67.

[53] Gadek JE, DeMichele SJ, Karlstad MD, et al. Effect of enteral feeding with eicosapentaenoic acid, gamma-linolenic acid, and antioxidants in patients with acute respiratory distress syndrome. Enteral Nutrition in ARDS Study Group. Crit Care Med 1999;27:1409–20.

[54] Nelson JL, DeMichele SJ, Pacht ER, et al. Effect of enteral feeding with eicosapentaenoic acid, gamma-linolenic acid, and antioxidants on antioxidant status in patients with acute respiratory distress syndrome. JPEN J Parenter Enteral Nutr 2003;27(2):98–104.

[55] Pacht ER, DeMichele SJ, Nelson JL, et al. Enteral nutrition with eicosapentaenoic acid, gamma-linolenic acid, and antioxidants reduces alveolar inflammatory mediators and protein influx in patients with acute respiratory distress syndrome. Crit Care Med 2003;31(2):491–500.

[56] Singer P, Theilla M, Fisher H, et al. Benefit of an enteral diet enriched with eicosapentaenoic acid and gamma-linolenic acid in ventilated patients with acute lung injury. Crit Care Med 2006;34(4):1033–8.

[57] Reisman J, Schachter HM, Dales RE, et al. Treating asthma with omega-3 fatty acids: where is the evidence? A systematic review. BMC Complement Altern Med 2006;6:26.

[58] Lekka ME, Liokatis S, Nathanail C, et al. The impact of intravenous fat emulsion administration in acute lung injury. Am J Respir Crit Care Med 2004;169(5):638–44.

[59] Kelly FJ. Vitamins and respiratory disease: antioxidant micronutrients in pulmonary health and disease. Proc Nutr Soc 2005;64:510–26.

[60] Barnes PJ. Reactive oxygen species and airway inflammation. Free Radic Biol Med 1990;9: 235–43.

[61] Turek JJ, Watkins BA, Schoenlein IA, et al. Oxidized lipid depresses canine growth, immune function, and bone formation. J Nutr Biochem 2003;14(1):24–31.

[62] Britton JR, Pavord I, Richards K, et al. Dietary antioxidant vitamin intake and lung function in the general population. Am J Respir Crit Care Med 1995;151:1383–7.

[63] McKeever TM, Britton J. Diet and asthma. Am J Respir Crit Care Med 2004;170: 725–9.

[64] Metnitz PG, Bartens C, Fischer M, et al. Antioxidant status in patients with acute respiratory distress syndrome. Intensive Care Med 1999;25(2):134–6.

[65] Nathens AB, Neff MJ, Jurkovich GJ, et al. Randomized, prospective trial of antioxidant supplementation in critically ill surgical patients. Ann Surg 2002;236:814–22.

[66] Schunemann HJ, McCann S, Grant BJ, et al. Lung function in relation to intake of carotenoids and other antioxidant vitamins in a population-based study. Am J Epidemiol 2002;155(5): 463–71.

[67] Shaheen SO, Sterne JA, Thompson RL, et al. Dietary antioxidants and asthma in animals. Am J Respir Crit Care Med 2001;164:1823–8.

[68] Steinmetz KA, Potter JD. Vegetables, fruit, and cancer. I. Epidemiology. Cancer Causes Control 1991;2:325–57.

[69] Troisi RJ, Willett WC, Weiss ST, et al. A prospective study of diet and adult-onset asthma. Am J Respir Crit Care Med 1995;151:1401–8.

[70] Wood LG, Fitzgerald DA, Lee AK, et al. Improved antioxidant and fatty acid status of patients with cystic fibrosis after antioxidant supplementation is linked to improved lung function. Am J Clin Nutr 2002;77:150–9.

[71] Repine JE, Bast A, Lankhorst I. Oxidative stress in chronic obstructive pulmonary disease. Oxidative Stress Study Group. Am J Respir Crit Care Med 1997;156:341–57.

[72] Becvarova I, Troy GC, Swecker WS Jr, et al. The effect of vitamin E enriched parenteral admixture on oxidative status of obese cats. Presented as an abstract at the 2005 Nestlé Purina Nutrition Forum; 2005.

[73] Droge W. Free radicals in the physiologic control of cell function. Physiol Rev 2002;82: 47–95.

[74] Ricciarelli R, Zingg JM, Azzi A. Vitamin E: protective role of a Janus molecule. FASEB J 2001;15:2314–25.

[75] Tucker JM, Townsend DM. Alpha-tocopherol: roles in prevention and therapy of human disease. Biomed Pharmacother 2005;59(7):380–7.

[76] Noverr MC, Huffnagle GB. The 'microflora hypothesis' of allergic diseases. Clin Exp Allergy 2005;35(12):1511–20.

[77] Schuller-Lewis GB, Sturman JA. Activation of alveolar leukocytes isolated from cats fed taurine-free diets. Adv Exp Med Biol 1992;315:83–90.

[78] Mawby DI, Bartges JM, DAvignon A, et al. Comparison of various methods for estimating body fat in dogs. J Am Anim Hosp Assoc 2004;40(2):109–14.

[79] Burkholder WJ, Bauer JE. Foods and techniques for managing obesity in companion animals. J Am Vet Med Assoc 1998;212(5):658–62.

[80] Butterwick RF, Hawthorne AJ. Advances in dietary management of obesity in dogs and cats. J Nutr 1998;128(12 Suppl):2771S–5S.

[81] German AJ. The growing problem of obesity in dogs and cats. J Nutr 2006;136(7 Suppl): 1940S–6S.

[82] Kealy RD, Lawler DF, Ballam JM, et al. Effects of diet restriction on life span and age-related changes in dogs. J Am Vet Med Assoc 2002;220(9):1315–20.

[83] Lawler DF, Evans RH, Larson BT, et al. Influence of lifetime food restriction on causes, time, and predictors of death in dogs. J Am Vet Med Assoc 2005;226(2):225–31.

[84] Yaissle JE, Holloway C, Buffington CA. Evaluation of owner education as a component of obesity treatment programs for dogs. J Am Vet Med Assoc 2004;224(12):1932–5.

[85] Bruchim Y, Klement E, Saragusty J, et al. Heat stroke in dogs: a retrospective study of 54 cases (1999–2004) and analysis of risk factors for death. J Vet Intern Med 2006;20(1):38–46.

[86] Dorsten CM, Cooker DM. Use of body condition scoring to manage body weight in dogs. Contemp Top Anim Sci 2004;43(3):34–7.

[87] Kulmatycki KM, Jamali F. Drug disease interactions: role of inflammatory mediators in disease and variability in drug response. J Pharm Pharm Sci 2005;8(3):602–25.

[88] Bernaerts F, Bolognin M, Dehard S, et al. Effect of obesity in dogs on airway reactivity measured by barometric whole body plethysmography. Presented at the 16th Congress of the European College of Veterinary Internal Medicine. Amsterdam, Netherlands, September 14–16, 2006.

[89] Bolognin M, Bernaerts F, Herpigny F, et al. Effect of obesity on doxapram hydrochloride-induced effects on whole body barometric plethysmography measurements in healthy beagle dogs. Presented at the 24th Symposium of the Veterinary Comparative Respiratory Society. Lena, Germany, October 8–10, 2006.

[90] LaFlamme DP. Understanding and managing obesity in dogs and cats. Vet Clin North Am Small Anim Pract 2006;36(6):1283–95.

[91] Olson AL, Zwillich C. The obesity hypoventilation syndrome. Am J Med 2005;118(9): 948–56.

[92] Poulain M, Doucet M, Major GC, et al. Pathophysiology and therapeutic strategies. CMAJ 2006;174(9):1293–9.

[93] Weitzenblum E, Kessler R, Chaouat A. Alveolar hypoventilation in the obese: the obesity-hypoventilation syndrome. Rev Pneumol Clin 2002;58(2):83–90.

[94] Wills J, Harvey R. Diagnosis and management of food allergy and intolerance in dogs and cats. Aust Vet J 1994;71(10):322–6.

[95] Poncet CM, Dupre GP, Freiche VG, et al. Long-term results of upper respiratory syndrome surgery and gastrointestinal tract medical treatment in 51 brachycephalic dogs. J Small Anim Pract 2006;47(3):137–42.

[96] Poncet CM, Dupre GP, Freiche VG, et al. Prevalence of gastrointestinal tract lesions in 73 brachycephalic dogs with upper respiratory syndrome. J Small Anim Pract 2005;46(6): 273–9.

INDEX

Note: Page numbers of article titles are in **boldface** type.

0195-5616/07/$ – see front matter
doi:10.1016/S0195-5616(07)00098-8

Moving?

Make sure your subscription moves with you!

To notify us of your new address, find your **Clinics Account Number** (located on your mailing label above your name), and contact customer service at:

E-mail: elspcs@elsevier.com

800-654-2452 (subscribers in the U.S. & Canada)
407-345-4000 (subscribers outside of the U.S. & Canada)

Fax number: 407-363-9661

Elsevier Periodicals Customer Service
6277 Sea Harbor Drive
Orlando, FL 32887-4800

*To ensure uninterrupted delivery of your subscription, please notify us at least 4 weeks in advance of move.